IMMUNIZATION IN PRACTICE

Facts & FAQs

IMMUNIZATION IN PRACTICE

Facts & FAQs

Mukesh Agrawal MD

Professor & Head (Ex)
Department of Pediatrics
Seth GS Medical College & KEM Hospital
Mumbai

Bhalani Publishers

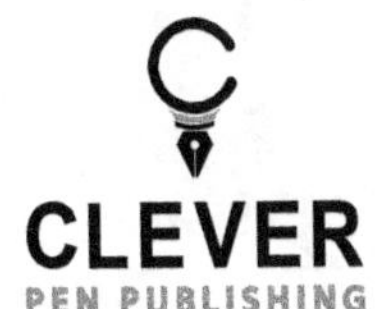

First Edition: 2022

This book has been published in good faith that the material provided by the author is a compilation of the original works done by great people. Every effort is made to ensure accuracy of the material, but the publisher, printer and author will not be held responsible for any inadvertent error(s). In case of any dispute, all legal matters will be settled under Mumbai jurisdiction only.

Published by:

BHALANI PUBLISHERS and
Clever Pen Publishing
(A joint venture between Bhalani Publishers and National Medical Book House)
D-2 Neelkanth Business Park Co-op. Premises Society Lt.
Nathani Road
Vidyavihar (West)
Mumbai 400086
Mob.: 09867214519

Email:
bhalanipublishers@gmail.com
cleverpen9@gmail.com

ISBN 978-93-92215-03-2

Printed & Bound in India

With lots of Love....

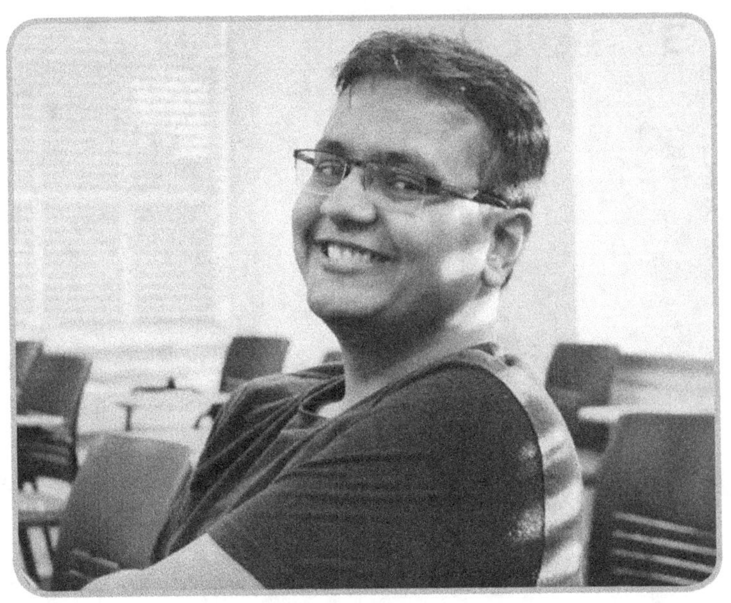

Ayush

Preface

Immunization is one of the greatest advances in medicine during last century, amply proven to reduce the disease, disability and death in children. Even if the eradication of smallpox in 1978 is an old story, two more recent milestones in India – elimination of Polio since 2014 and Maternal & Neonatal Tetanus since 2015, underscore immense value of Immunization in the public health. None to forget the role, Covid-19 vaccines are playing globally, to control the ongoing pandemic.

Vaccinology is a rapidly advancing science with every day something being added to our knowledge and practice. At present, reasonably safe and effective vaccines are available for over 25 diseases and about 500 plus products are in pipeline against additional diseases or as alternatives to existing products. To update this knowledge and use it in practice is a big challenge. Moreover, immunization needs of each child might be different from others and require logical modifications in the practice.

While many excellent resources in the print and electronic media are available on vaccines and immunization, most of them are usually too exhaustive. Present book aims to provide state-of-the-art information in a simple and concise format and to answer frequently faced dilemma in immunization practice. While specially targeting practicing pediatricians and undergraduate students, this book is also expected to be a good primer for postgraduates.

I am indebted to my colleagues and students who pushed me to take up this project and complete in time. My family too has been a constant support in this endeavor, always encouraging to accept such challenges.

I also wish to place on record my appreciation to the Mr. Rajesh Bhalani and Mr. Rushabh Bhalani from Bhalani Publishers and Mrs. Harsha Shah from National Medical Book House for the excellent production work along with the DTP typesetter for his print-setting skills.

Corrections, suggestions, feedback and reviews are welcome from readers to improve further edition, which may be sent at *dr_mukesh_agrawal@yahoo.co.in*

Dr. Mukesh Agrawal
Professor & Head (Ex)
Department of Pediatrics
Seth GS Medical College & KEM Hospital
Mumbai

Abbreviations

AEFI	:	Adverse Event Following Immunization
AIDS	:	Acquired Immunodeficiency Syndrome
ARV	:	Anti-Rabies vaccine
B	:	Booster
BCG:	:	Bacillus calmette Guerin
DPT	:	Diptheria, Pertusis & Tetanus vaccine
DT	:	Diptheria & Pertusis vaccine
DTwP	:	Diphtheria, Tetanus & whole cell Pertusis vaccine
DTaP	:	Diphtheria, Tetanus & acellular Pertusis vaccine
FAQ	:	Frequently Asked Questions
fIPV	:	fractionated Inactivated Polio Vaccine
GBS	:	Guillain Barre syndrome
HAV	:	Hepatitis A vaccine
HIV	:	Human Immunodeficiency virus
HBIG	:	Hepatitis B Immunoglobulin
HBV	:	Hepatitis B Vaccine
HDCV	:	Human Diploid Cell Vaccine
HHE	:	Hypotonic- Hyporesponsive Episodes
HIB	:	Hemophilus influenzae B vaccine
HiB	:	Hemophilus influenzae B virus
HPV	:	Human Papillomavirus Vaccine
IAP	:	Indian Academy of Pediatrics
Ig	:	Immunoglobulin
IIV	:	Inactivated Influenza Vaccine
IM	:	Intramuscular
IPV	:	Inactivated Polio Vaccine
IVIG	:	Intravenous immunoglobulins
JE	:	Japanese Encephalitis
Mab	:	Monoiclonal antibodies
MCV	:	Meningococcal conjugate vaccine
Mo	:	Month
MPSV	:	Meningococcal Polysaccharide vaccine
MR	:	Measles & Rubella Vaccine
MMR	:	Measles, Mumps & Rubella Vaccine

MMRV	:	Measles, Mumps, Rubella & Varicella vaccine
NIS	:	National Immunization schedule
OPV	:	Oral Polio Vaccine
PCV	:	Pneumococcal Conjugate vaccine
PCEV	:	Purified Chick Embryo Vaccine
PDEV	:	Purified Duck Embryo Vaccine
PentaV	:	Pentavalent Vaccine (DTwP+HIB+HBV)
PEP	:	Post-Exposure Prophylaxis
PO	:	Per oral
PPI	:	Pulse Polio Immunization
PPSV	:	Pneumococcal Polysaccharide vaccine
PrEP	:	Pre-Exposure Prophylaxis
PVRV	:	Purified Verocell Rabies vaccine
RIG	:	Rabies Immunoglobulin
RV	:	Rotavirus Vaccine
SC	:	Subcutaneous
TCV	:	Typhoid Conjugate vaccine
Td	:	Tetanus & Diphtheria (Low-dose) vaccine
TdaP	:	Tetanus,Diphtheria (Low-dose) & acellular Pertusis vaccine
TPSV	:	Typhoid Polysaccharide disease
TT	:	Tetanus Toxoid
UIP	:	Universal Immunization Program
VAPP	:	Vaccine Associated Paralytic Poliomyelitis
VCZ	:	Varicella Zoster
VDPV	:	Vaccine Derived Polio Virus
WHO	:	World Health organization
Wk	:	Week
YFV	:	Yellow fever vaccine
Yr	:	Year

CONTENTS

Feedback

Help Us Improve

Scan the QR code
and give your feedback
Or
You can email us your feedback on
☞ bhalanipublishers@gmail.com
☞ cleverpen9@gmail.com

Section

I

General Considerations

Physiological Concepts in Immunology

Initial host-defense mechanisms against invasion by a pathogen include - (a) *anatomical integrity of* skin and mucosal membranes, (b) *physiological milieu* of the tissues e.g. acidic gastric pH to prevent local survival and growth, (c) *mechanical clearance* of pathogens and cell debris, e.g. mucociliary movements, and (d) competitive opposition against localization of pathogens by *normal microbial colonizing flora.* Once these barriers are breached, second line of defense involves *immunological system –* a complex interplay of various components acting in unison to eliminate the invading pathogen *or* even an aberrant host-antigen, e.g. tumor cells.

1.1: IMMUNITY

The term *immunity* refers to *complete protection or at least partial resistance against an infection,* provided by two major defense mechanisms - Innate immunity and Adaptive or acquired immunity (**Table 1.1**).

Innate immunity denotes the protective mechanisms present since birth which are *antigen non-specific* and attempts to eliminate any invading pathogen immediately on exposure, before the development of specific adaptive immunity. Innate immunity is provided by – *a) Physical, chemical and mechanical barriers* enumerated earlier, *b) Inflammatory response* to bring cellular elements at the site of invasion and increase lymphatic flow to move microbes and antigen-bearing cells towards the lymphoid tissue, c) *Cellular components* e.g. phagocytes and Natural killer cells to engulf and kill invading organisms, and d) release of chemical mediators e.g. cytokines and chemokines.

Table 1.1: Innate *vs* Adaptive Immunity		
	Innate immunity	**Adaptive immunity**
Specificity	Antigen Non-specific	Antigen Specific
Acts..	Immediately after exposure	Develops after few days
Longevity	Short-lasting, No memory	Long-lasting, memory develops
Protectivity	More important during first exposure	More important during subsequent exposures
Mediators:		
a. Cellular	Phagocytes*	T-helper cells
	Dendritic cells	Naïve B- cells
	Natural killer T- cells	Memory- B cells
b. Humoral	Complement	Immunoglobulins
	Cytokines & Chemokines	
	Acute Phase reactants	

* Neutrophils, Macrophages and monocytes

Innate immune system also triggers development of adaptive immunity by processing the pathogen by *antigen presenting cells or APCs* (Macrophages and Dendritic cells). APCs engulf the pathogen, express their antigens on the cell surface and transport them to T-Lymphocytes, largely present in lymph nodes. Vaccines which also stimulate innate immunity are better immunogens.

Adaptive immunity is second line of immunological defense which is *antigen-specific*. It develops after few days of exposure and persists throughout the life, though not necessarily in the protective range. Adaptive immunity plays a major role not only in clearance of primary infection but also in prevention of disease during subsequent exposure by developing the Immunological memory. It is mediated by T-lymphocytes or T-cells *(Cell-mediated immunity)* and/or B-lymphocytes or B-cells generated immunoglobulins *(Humoral immunity)*.

Cell-mediated immunity is the principal defense against *intracellular pathogens,* mainly involving T-cells. T-cells can not recognize the microorganisms unless presented by APCs as processed antigens (epitopes). T-cell receptors bind to these epitopes and differentiate into *T-helper* and *T-cytotoxic* cells. T-helper cells secrete *cytokines to* simulate proliferation and differentiation of B lymphocytes for antibody production. Cytotoxic T-cells recognize and kill infected cells directly by lysis or by secreting specific cytokines. T-cell responses are more robust, long-lasting, and cross-protective than humoral responses. Another set of regulatory T-cells, termed as *T-Suppressor cells* and control the immune response to keep the immune system from becoming over-active.

Humoral immunity is the principal defense mechanism against *extracellular pathogens and toxins,* mediated through antibodies of various classes e.g. IgG, IgM, IgA etc. These antibodies are secreted by B-lymphocytes or B-cells in Biological fluids (*humors,* hence the term Humoral). B-cells have immunoglobulin molecules (antibodies) on their surface membranes, which act as receptors (paratopes) for the antigens. These antibody receptors bind either to T-helper cells activated by APCs (*T-cell dependent response*) or directly to extracellular microorganisms e.g. bacteria (*T-cell independent response*).

Each antibody can recognize and bind to only one specific antigen. Once an antigen binds to the specific antibody-receptor, B-cell differentiates into plasma cells *or* memory cells. Plasma cells operate as factories to manufacture and secrete specific antibodies, which eliminate the pathogen by processes of neutralization, opsonization or complement-activation. Antibodies also inhibit local colonization by pathogens. B-memory cells remain at rest till re-exposure, when they trigger rapid anamnestic response to produce large quantity of antibodies (*Immunological memory*).

T-cell dependent vs T-cell independent response:

Most of the antigens produce *T-cell dependent response* using APCs > T-Helper cells > B-cells > Plasma cells > antibodies and

Memory cells route. These antigens are termed as T-cell dependent antigens and antibodies against them are primarily of IgG class. T-cell dependent response also produces memory-B cells for robust anamnestic response on re-exposure.

T-cell independent response is usually seen against the organisms covered by a polysaccharide capsule (e.g. HiB, Pneumococci, meningococci). This capsule resists ingestion of organism by phagocytes, preventing expression of antigen and T-cell activation. In such cases, naïve B cells themselves recognize the pathogen and get activated to produce antibodies. Antibodies produced against T-cell independent responses are largely of IgM class, and no memory cells develop for anamnestic response on re-exposure.

Figure 1.1 presents a schematic representation of important immune responses following exposure to a pathogen.

1.2 : IMMUNIZATION

Depending on the mode of acquisition, Immunity may also be broadly classified as *Active* acquired after exposure to foreign antigen/s through natural infection or vaccination or *Passive* acquired through transplacentally transferred antibodies or administration of pre-formed immunoglobulins in later life. Active immunity does not provide instant protection and takes few days to develop but persists for many years, once acquired. On the other side, Passive immunity provides instant protection on exposure but last only for few weeks.

The term Immunization denotes the induction of specific immune response by either - a) deliberate inoculation of antigens stimulate *in vivo* antibody production (*active immunization or vaccination*), or b) administration of pre-formed antibodies, i.e. immunoglobulins (*passive immunization*).

Although frequently used interchangeably, the terms *immunization* and *vaccination* have different connotations. Vaccination denotes *a process to administer antigen/s for active*

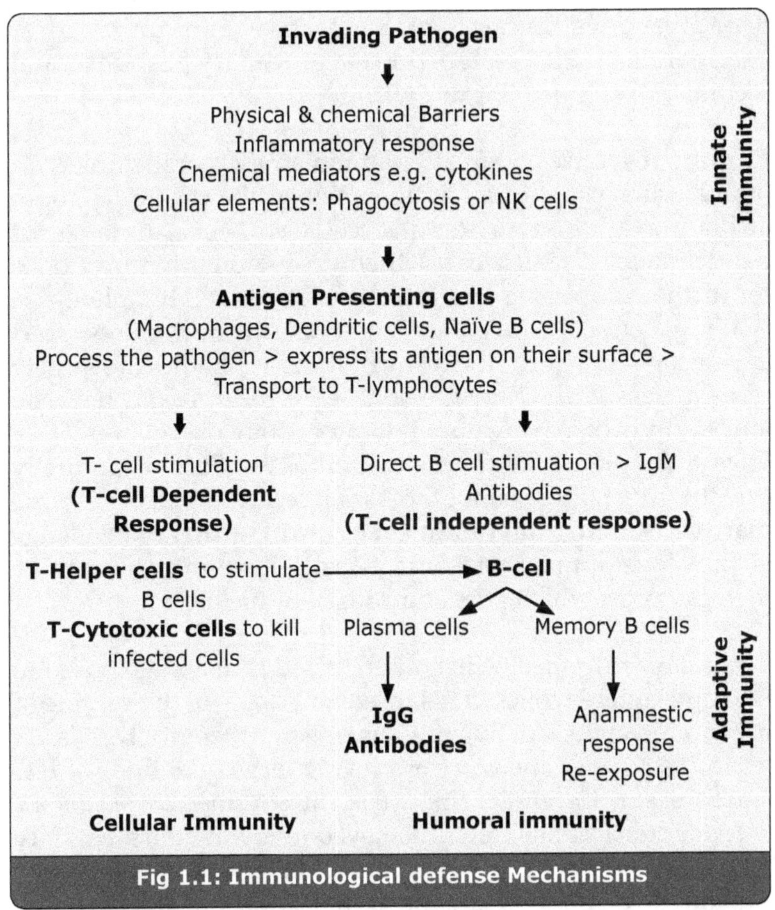

Fig 1.1: Immunological defense Mechanisms

immunization, excluding passive immunization. Moreover, a vaccinated child may not essentially be considered as immunized, if the desired immune response is not induced due to any reason including faulty vaccine, faulty technique or immunocompromized host.

Primary objective of the vaccination is *to trigger and sustain disease-specific immune response above the protective threshold*, by exposing the immune system to deliberately introduce antigen/s devoid of pathogenic properties i.e. vaccine. This response may be either *humoral* with antibody production, or *cellular* with T-cell activation or *both*.

Broadly, development of protective immunity after vaccination is a two-step process—primary response and secondary response (**Figure 1.2**).

Primary response: Soon after administration of the first dose of a vaccine, constituent antigen/s elicit the innate response attracting antigen processing cells e.g. macrophages or dendritic cells, which carry them to regional lymph nodes for further processing and activation of T and B lymphocytes. After about 3-5 days, antigen-specific antibodies start appearing in the serum. However, these antibodies are largely of IgM class with short life-span (21–28 days) and have no long-term protective value. IgG titers start rising after 21-28 days and remain high for many months but decline gradually due to short life span of plasma cells outside the bone marrow. Another important event during primary challenge is the development of some B cells into antigen-specific memory cells, which persist throughout the life.

Secondary response: When a sensitized host is re-exposed to the same antigen following subsequent doses of the vaccine or natural infection, existing antigen-specific memory B-cells are rapidly activated and start producing large quantities of IgG antibodies by the end of first week , also termed as *anamnestic or booster response*. IgG titers achieved following the secondary response are not only high quantitatively but also remain sustained for many years since many plasma cells by now reach survival niches in the bone marrow and continue to produce antibodies. These high and sustained IgG antibodies are protective for many years or for life. IgM response on re-exposure, though occurs, is less pronounced and short-lived. In cases of non-replicating inactivated or sub-unit vaccines or toxoids, development of adequately protective antibody levels after vaccination requires at least two exposures at different time intervals – first one is termed as the priming dose and subsequent dose as the booster dose. Some vaccines may need more than one priming doses or booster doses. Usually a minimal interval of 3 weeks is required between multiple primary doses to allow development of successive

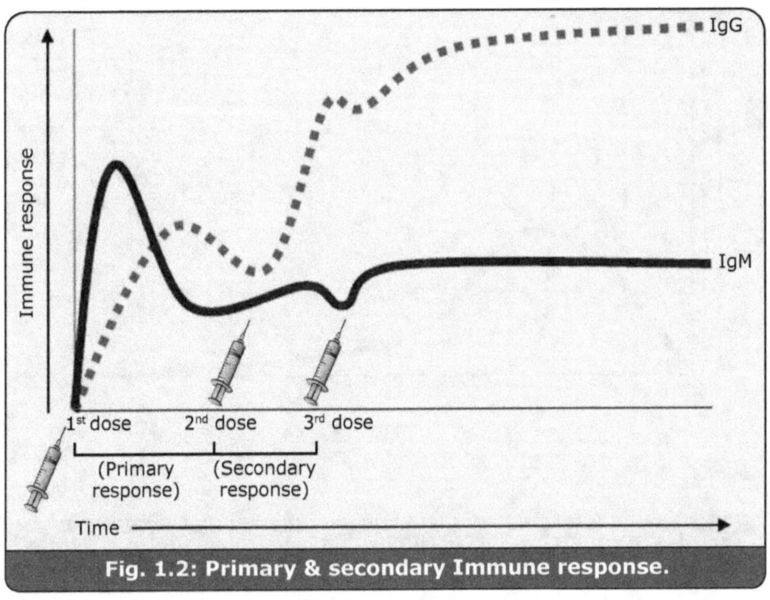

Fig. 1.2: Primary & secondary Immune response.

waves of Ag-specific primary responses without interference, while a minimum Interval of 4 months is required between priming and boosting doses to allow affinity maturation of memory B cells and thus higher secondary responses (**Figure 1.2**)

However, in case of live vaccines, *in vivo* replication of organisms provide a sustained source of antigen for longer periods, leading to merging of the primary and secondary immune responses. Hence, booster doses are usually not required for live vaccines, though given in some cases to enhance the coverage (**Figure 1.3**).

Most of the vaccines mediate protective efficacy through production of disease-specific IgG antibodies, though live vaccines also generate strong protective response through CD8+ cytotoxic T cells. Newer vaccines have started using live vectors as vehicle to induce strong CD8+ T-cell responses.

Polysaccharides are poor antigens and early-generation poly-saccharide vaccines usually produce T-cell independent re-

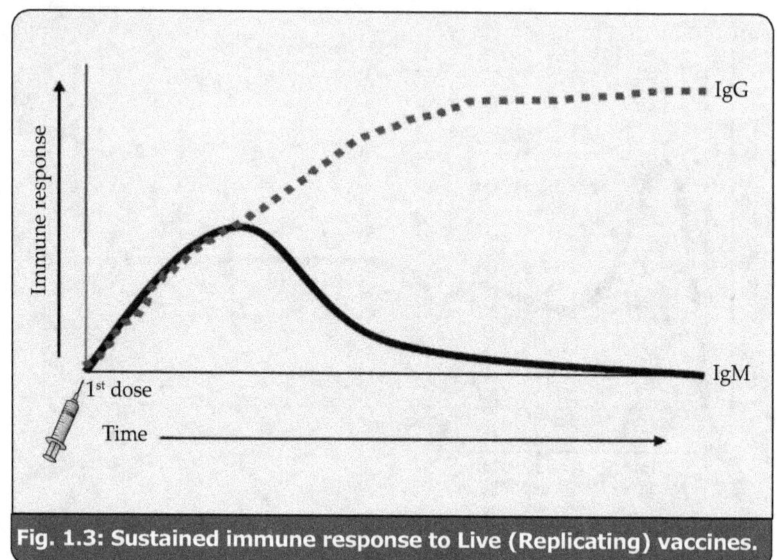

Fig. 1.3: Sustained immune response to Live (Replicating) vaccines.

sponse, which is largely of IgM class with no development of memory cells. To overcome these handicaps, polysaccharide antigens are now usually conjugated with a protein carrier (e.g. Toxoid) to produce strong IgG response and memory cells.

Induction of antigen-specifc antibodies or other immune responses by an immunization process does not necessarily imply that these responses could be taken as correlates of protection and need to be confirmed by clinical trials.

Frequently Asked Questions (FAQs)

1.   **What is an Antigen?**

Antigen is a molecule capable of stimulating an immune response in the body, which may be a foreign substance e.g. viruses, bacteria, toxins, and parasites or even an aberrant host-antigen, e.g. tumor cells. Each antigen has distinct surface features which are recognized by specific cells of the immune system.

2. What is an antibody?

Antibodies, also known as Immunoglobulins (Ig) are large Y-shaped protein used by immune system, with five main classes - IgM, IgG, IgA, IgD and IgE. Of these, first three are involved in immunization process, while IgE is a mediator of allergy and IgD has no definite activity except being an antigen receptor on the surfaces of B cells.

IgM are first antibodies to appear following Antigenic exposure (~3-5 days) but have a short life of only ~21-28 days. These antibodies act in initial phases of infection by complement activation and lysis of cells with a limited role in protection against the infection. However, elevated antigen-specific IgM levels are important diagnostic markers of recent infection. IgM antibodies do not cross the placenta.

IgG, principal humoral component of immune defense, constitutes ~80% of serum antibodies. These antibodies appear after ~3-4 weeks (earlier in case of re-exposure) and remain high for a long time. IgG are only antibodies to cross the placenta and protect newborn. Elevated antigen-specific IgG antibodies are indicators of past infection, more useful markers for epidemiologists but of limited use for diagnosis of acute infection.

IgA constitutes only 10-20% of serum antibodies but present in large amounts in tissues to block the attachment of pathogens on mucosal surfaces. These antibodies also protect against enterotoxins e.g. cholera and eliminate food antigens. IgA are also present in abundance in secretions e.g. breast milk, saliva, tears, respiratory and digestive secretions etc.

3. What is epitope and paratope?

Epitope is the part of the antigen which is recognized by the immune system, while *Paratope* is the part of the antibody that recognizes the corresponding epitope.

4. **What are antigenic-Processing cells and how do they function?**

Antigenic presenting cells (APCs) are the cells which can't kill the bacteria themselves but engulf them and express the bacterial antigen on their surface, to render them recognizable by T cells for elimination. These cells include Dendritic cells in tissues, Macrophages in circulation and tissues both, and Naive B cell in circulation.

5. **What are T- cells and B-cells, also termed as T- and B-lymphocytes?**

T- Lymphocytes are like the *orchestra director* for acquired immunity, which not only mediate cellular immunity but also activate B-cells for immunoglobulin production. These cells develop in the bone marrow, but later migrate and mature in thymus before re-populating lymphoid organs. Depending on their functions and CD markers, T cells are divided into - *a) T helper cells* (CD4+cells), which induce antibody production by B cells and regulate immune response by cytokines production *and b) Cytotoxic-suppressor cells* (CD8+ cells), responsible for killing of virus-infected cells *or* tumor cells directly or through specific cytokines. Another set of Regulatory T-cells (T- Suppressor cells) suppress lymphocytes and control the immune response

B-lymphocytes are the source of antibodies, which on receiving the antigenic stimulus, differentiate into plasma cells and produce immunoglobulins. B-cells develop and mature in bone marrow itself (unlike T-cells, which mature in thymus) before populating lymphoid follicles. B-cells are of two types - B1 cells (CD5+ cells), which produce non-specific IgM immunoglobulins against variety of antigens; and B2 cells which produce antigen-specific antibodies.

6. **What is Th-1 and Th-2 cells?**

T-helper cells were initially used to be divided into - *Th1 cells* important for macrophage activation and cell-mediated immunity; and *Th2 cells,* which help in activation and differentiation of B cells and down-regulation of immune response. However, with identification of many more subsets of Th cells, this classification is largely outdated. Currently, main subsets include– a) Follicular T-helper (Tfh) cells involved in B cell activation and differentiation into antibody producing plasma cells; b) Th1 cells mainly involved in protection against intracellular pathogens (viruses, Mycobacterium tuberculosis); c) Th2 and Th9 cells respond to extracellular pathogens (bacteria and helminths) and d) Th17 cells which contribute to mucosal defense, specially against respiratory pathogens.

7. **What is Memory cells?**

Memory cells are B-lymphocytes which develop along with plasma cells in response to a T cell - dependent antigen but do not participate in immune process and remain as resting cells. However, on re-exposure to the same antigen, these cells rapidly proliferate and differentiate into plasma cells to secrete large quantity of specific antibodies (*Anamnestic response*).

8. **What is the difference between T cell- dependent and T cell- independent antigens?**

Most of the antigens require T helper cells to stimulate B cells for antibody production and are referred as *T cell-dependent* antigens. Antibodies against T cell-dependent antigens are primarily of IgG class and the response also produces memory B cells for robust anamnestic response on re-exposure.

However in some cases, specially when the organism is covered with a polysaccharide capsule (e.g. Hemophilus influenzae B, Pneumococci, meningococci) which resists ingestion by phagocytes and avoid T-cell stimulation, B cells can produce antibodies directly, without the help of T cells. However, antibodies produced against such antigens are of IgM class and immunologic memory is not created.

9. How do antibodies eliminate antigens?

Antibodies eliminate the pathogens by three major mechanisms – a) *Neutralization* i.e. binding pathogens to block their access to cells which are then engulfed and cleared by macrophages; b) *Opsonization*: Encapsulated organisms which are not directly recognized by the macrophages or dendritic cells and evade the innate immune system are recognized by antibodies. These antibodies coat them to enable the ingestion by macrophages and dendritic cells through the process of opsonization,; and c) *Complement Activation*: Antibodies also bind to certain bacteria in the plasma as well as complements to lyse the bacteria or attract the macrophages to it.

10. Whether the terms "immunization" and "vaccination" are same?

Although frequently used interchangeably, the terms *immunization* and *vaccination* have different connotations. *Vaccination* denotes a *process* to administer immunogenic agents i.e. vaccines for active immunization, while *Immunization* refers to the actual induction of specific immune response following vaccination. A vaccinated child may not be truly immunized, if the immunological response failed to develop due to some reason.

References

1. Pollard, A.J et al. A guide to vaccinology: from basic principles to new developments. Nat Rev Immunol 2021, 21; 83–100.
2. World Health Organization. Vaccine Immunology. Available from: https://www.who.int/immunization/documents/Elsevier_Vaccine_immunology.pdf (accessed on July 11,2021).
3. Pemde H et al. Basic Immunology. *In*: IAP Guidebook on Immunization 2018-19 - Advisory Committee on Vaccines and Immunization Practices, Indian Academy of Pediatrics, 3rd Edition, New Delhi, Jaypee Brothers 2020, pp 14-27.
4. Paul Y et al. Vaccine Immunology – Basics and Beyond. *In*: Vashishtha V et al. FAQs on Vaccines and immunization practices. 2nd Edition. New Delhi, Jaypee Brothers 2015, pp 3-24.
5. Agrawal M. Immunity and Immunological disorders. *In*: Agrawal M. Textbook of Pediatrics. 2nd ed. New Delhi: CBS Publishers, 2017, pp 118-132.

Immunization Agents (Vaccines)

Immunization agents are biological products to provide or provoke immunity when introduced into the body *and include both – those to provide passive immunity e.g. Immunoglobulins* and antisera etc, and those to provoke active immunity e.g. vaccines. Passive immunization agents introduce preformed IgG antibodies for immediate but short-lasting protection, more suited for post-exposure prophylaxis. This chapter mainly deals with active immunization agents i.e. vaccines, which provide relatively slower but more robust and sustained immune response.

Vaccines are formulations containing live attenuated or inactivated pathogens, their subunits or toxins, retaining the antigenic properties but devoid of the virulence. In addition to the main antigen/s, these formulations also include variety of other ingredients (Excipients) to e.g. Adjuvants, Preservatives, stabilizers etc to enhance the immunogenicity or stability of the vaccines.

2.1: TYPES OF VACCINES

Currently available vaccines may be classified into different types based upon the viability of organisms and characteristics of the antigenic components (**Table 2.1**).

Depending on the number of antigens, vaccines may also be termed as *Monovalent* i.e. containing a single strain of the organism e.g. Measles or *Polyvalent* vaccines containing two or more strains of same organism e.g. bivalent OPV. Vaccines which contain antigens from two or more organisms are termed as *combination vaccines* e.g. MMR or DPT (Sec 2.3)

Table 2.1: Common types of Vaccines	
I. Live vaccines	
Bacterial	BCG
Viral	OPV, RV, MR/MMR, Varicella, JE, Yellow Fever
II. Inactivated vaccines	
Bacterial	Pertussis (Whole cell), Cholera
Viral	IPV, HAV, HBV, HPV, JE (Inactivated) , Influenza
III. Toxoids	Diphtheria, Tetanus
IV. Subunit vaccines	
Protein	Pertussis (acellular)
Polysachharide	PPSV, MPSV, TPSV
Conjugated	HIB, TCV, PCV, MCV

OPV: Oral polio vaccine; **RV:** Rotavirus vaccine, **MR:** Measles & Rubella Vaccine, **MMR:** Measles, Mumps, Rubella vaccine; LAVI (Live attenuated A vaccine), **IPV:** Inactivated polio vaccine; **HBV:** Hepatitis B vaccine; **HAV:** Hepatitis A vaccine; **HPV:** Human Papillomavirus vaccine, **JE:** Japanese encephalitis vaccine; **HIB:** H. influenzae B vaccine, **MPSV:** Meningococcal polysaccharide vaccine, **PPSV:** Pneumococcal Polysaccharide vaccine; **TPSV:** Typhoid Polysaccharide vaccine, **TCV:** Typhoid Conjugate vaccine, **PCV:** Pneumococcal conjugate vaccine, **MCV:** Meningococcal Conjugate vaccine.

Live vaccines contain viable organisms - bacteria or viruses, which have been *attenuated* or weakened during the manufacturing process to reduce their virulence, though still retaining some ability to replicate in the host and provoke immune response. These attenuated strains are developed either by passing the virulent organism through a series of cell cultures under sub-optimal conditions or modifying/deleting their virulence genes by recombinant technology.

Major advantage of live vaccines is that they are highly immunogenic. Endogenous replication of inoculated organism mimics natural infection with - a) more sustained supply of antigen and b) stimulation of both humoral as well as cell-mediated immunity. Immunity after these vaccines is robust, long-lasting if not life-long, and boosters are rarely required barring few exceptions. In fact, the secondary response on revaccination with live vaccines might be blunted due to presence of pre-existing antibodies, which neutralize the vaccine virus.

Major disadvantages of live vaccines include - a) Need for stringent storage conditions to maintain the viability of organisms, b) Contraindication to use in Immunocompromized persons, c) Potential risk of reverting to virulence leading to vaccine associated disease e.g. Vaccine associated paralytic poliomyelitis (VAPP), Very rarely, live vaccines grown in large quantities in culture vessels might get contaminated during the manufacturing process e.g. Monkey virus SV40 was detected in some preparations of the Sabin polio vaccine attenuated by passage through monkey kidney cells.

More than one live vaccines, if necessary, have to be given together on the same day or at least with 28 days interval since developing immune response to the first inoculation may affect the response to subsequent vaccine.

Inactivated (Killed) vaccines contain whole-cell organisms, inactivated using heat or chemicals e.g. Formaldehyde to destroy their capability to replicate and cause disease. These products retain their immunogenicity but with limited antigenic load due to no endogenous replication.

Main disadvantage of inactivated vaccines is that these are poorly immunogenic after the first dose and need multiple doses for the desired response. First dose acts as *priming dose* to initiate the production of memory B cells, which trigger pronounced anamnestic response to further doses. Moreover, immune response to an inactivated vaccine is largely humoral with little or no development of cellular immunity. Antibody titers wane over time and may require periodic booster doses for sustained protection.

Major advantage of inactivated vaccines is that these are - a) relatively heat and light stable and do not need very stringent storage conditions, and b) can be safely used in immunocompromised children.

Unlike live vaccines, response to inactivated antigens is usually not affected by circulating antibodies and hence, these vaccines can be given at any time interval with other vaccines or natural infections.

Although toxoids and subunit vaccines, discussed later, are also inactivated vaccines, the term is generally used to denote whole-cell inactivated vaccines only.

Toxoids: Some bacterial diseases are not directly caused by the pathogen but by a toxin produced by it e.g. Diphtheria or Tetanus. Toxoid vaccines are produced by neutralizing culprit toxins using heat or chemical e.g. Formalin to remove its toxicity. Immune response of these vaccines is targeted against the toxin and not *per se* the pathogen. Being non-replicating vaccines, these vaccines also need multiple doses and booster shots for adequate and sustained protection.

Sub-unit Vaccines: Subunit vaccines contain only selected antigens of a pathogen which are considered essential to stimulate immune response rather than the whole organism, thus providing desired immune response without the risk of disease.

Subunit vaccines are produced by – a) isolating specific antigen/s from the whole organism grown on culture e.g. acellular pertussis or Inactivated Influenza vaccines; or b) using recombinant technology in which a gene coding the desired antigenic protein is inserted into another virus or producer cells in culture to manufacture desired antigen in large amounts.

Depending on the constituent antigen, Subunit vaccines may be further classified as - a) *Protein-based* e.g. acellular pertussis or HBV vaccines or b) *Polysaccharide vaccines* e.g. in Pneumococcal and Meningococcal vaccines.

Polysaccharide vaccines use a specific component of the organism, e.g. polysaccharides of the bacterial cell wall or capsule as the antigen. Since these antigens are non-protein, Polysaccharide vaccines are poorly immunogenic with three main issues - a) highly inadequate immune response in children below 2 years of age due to immaturity of the marginal zones of spleen/nodes, where antigens binds B cells to differentiate them in plasma cells for antibody production, b) Antibody response of predominantly IgM class with lower and rapidly declining IgG titers, c) No T-cell response and no production of memory B cells, thus lack of anamnestic response on re-exposure.

Subsequent re-exposure to the same polysaccharide antigen results in a repeat primary response, again with low antibody titers, which decline rapidly. In fact, Revaccination with polysaccharide vaccines may induce even further lower antibody responses than the first dose, a phenomenon termed as the *immunological hyporesponsiveness*. Hence, these vaccines are sparingly used only in children above two years of age and more than two doses are generally not recommended.

Conjugated vaccines are modified polysaccharide vaccines in which component polysaccharide/s are conjugated with some other potent antigen, termed *vehicle* (e.g. mutant diphtheria or tetanus toxoid), to behave like inactivated T-cell dependent vaccines with better immunogenicity. Initial response to conjugate vaccines is similar to that with polysaccharide vaccines but some of the antigen-bind B cells migrate to germinal centers for more intense proliferation, differentiation into plasma cells and secrete large amount of antibodies. Few plasma cells also migrate to survival niches e.g. bone marrow, with prolonged persistence of antibodies. Development of memory B cells lead to anamnestic response of re-exposure. Unlike polysaccharide vaccines, conjugated vaccines can be used in younger children below 2 years of age and produce strong immune response including immune memory. However, like other inactivated vaccines, conjugated vaccines also require multiple doses for adequate and sustained immune response.

2.2: VACCINE EXCIPIENTS

In addition to biologically active antigen, vaccine formulations also contain many other additives e.g. adjuvants, preservatives, stabilizers, vehicle and diluents, collectively also termed as *Excipients*. These are immunologically inactive substances present in the final vaccine product (other than antigen), which are added for a specific purpose during the manufacturing processes. Some other substances are also added during the production but removed subsequently, though traces of them may be left behind in the final product. Excipients are responsible for some of the allergic reactions or adverse events attributed to the vaccine.

Adjuvants are pharmacological additives in some of the inactivated vaccines, specially subunit vaccines, to enhance the immunogenicity by permitting slower but more sustained delivery of antigens, attraction of immunocompetent cells around the injection site and modulation of Th responses to support or limit antibody production. However, presence of an adjuvant may also increase the incidence of local side-effects of a vaccine e.g. sterile abscess, nodules, granuloma or contact hypersensitivity.

Aluminium salts e.g. hydroxide, phosphate etc. have been used since long as adjuvants and many other newer adjuvants have been developed for use in modern vaccines, which target specific components of the body's immune response.

As a general rule, nearly all bacterial vaccines and Hepatitis A & B vaccines contain adjuvants, while most of the viral vaccines e.g. MMR, Varicella, Influenza etc. are adjuvant free, barring few exceptions.

Preservatives are added to inactivate pathogens or detoxify toxins during manufacturing and to prevent bacterial or fungal contamination on storage, specially in multi-dose vials. Vaccine which do not contain a preservative e.g. Measles, are associated with severe septic reactions, e.g. Toxic-shock syndrome, if used beyond 4-6 hours of reconstitution. Although present in very miniscule amount, these agents have been implicated in some allergic reactions or adverse events of vaccines.

Commonly used preservatives include mercurial compounds e.g., Thiomersal, antibiotics e.g. Neomycin and Formalde-hyde.

Stabilizers are largely used to maintain the potency of vaccine during storage, specially when the cold chain is unreliable. Apart from inappropriate temperature, Vaccines may also lose potency due to manufacturing process e.g. Freeze-drying, pH variations and adherence of antigen to glass vials. Bacterial vaccines can also become unstable on storage due to hydrolysis and aggregation of protein and carbohydrate molecules.

Commonly used stabilizers include magnesium chloride (for OPV), magnesium sulfate (for measles), lactose, sorbitol, Gelatin and albumin.

Diluents: Lyophilized (Freeze-dried) vaccines need to be reconstituted by dissolving in a diluents, before the administration. Only the diluents recommended by the manufacturer and supplied with the vaccine should be used for this purpose. Moreover, the expiry date of diluents must be checked separately, which might be different than that of the vaccine. Most of these vaccines are less stable after reconstitution and have to be used within few hours.

While sterile water is the most commonly used diluent for childhood vaccines, Normal saline is used for reconstitution of BCG, HIB (Some) and Yellow fever vaccines. Calcium carbonate and Citrated Sodium bicarbonate are specific diluents for lyophilized Rotavirus vaccines RV1 (Rotarix®) and BRV-PV (Rotasiil®) respectively.

2.3: COMBINATION VACCINES

Combination vaccines are vaccines containing antigenic material from different organisms e.g. DPT, DT, MMR and others (**Table 2.2**). These vaccines are useful to minimize the hospital visits, cost and number of pricks, improving the acceptance and compliance. IAP encourages use of combination vaccines for childhood immunization over separate injections of component vaccines.

Two major concerns with use of combination vaccines are - a) immunological interference between component antigens or excipients to affect the immunogenicity, and b) Cumulatively higher risk of adverse events.

Table 2.2. Combination vaccines available in India	
Number of Antigens	**Combination**
Bivalent (Two Antigen) Vaccines	DT or Td*
	MR*
	HAV+HBV
Trivalent (Three Antigen) Vaccines	DTwP, DTaP
	MMR
Quadrivalent (Four antigen) Vaccines	DTwP+HIB
	DTwP+HBV
	DTaP+IPV
	MMRV
Pentavalent (Five antigen) Vaccines	DTwP+HBV+HIB*
	DTaP+HBV+HIB
Hexavalent (Six antigen) vaccines	DTwP+HBV+HIB+IPV
	DTaP+HBV+HIB+IPV

* - Used in National Immunization schedule

However, there is no evidence that administration of several antigens in combined vaccines overwhelms the immune system, which has the capability of responding to millions of antigens at a time. All combination vaccines are licensed only after ensuring that efficacy of each antigenic component is comparable to respective stand-alone vaccines.

Similarly, the concern about cumulative risk of adverse events has not been substantiated in practice. In fact, combination vaccines might be associated with overall reduction in adverse reactions due to lesser number of injections.

However, some facts are worth remembering while using combination vaccines –

a) Total number of doses for combination vaccine should not be less than total number of doses recommended for each component antigen e.g. Instead of two doses of stand-alone HAV, three dose are needed, when given as HAV+HBV combination vaccine (Twinrix) since HBV is a minimum three-dose vaccine.

b) Minimum interval between two doses of combination vaccines should not be less than the recommended for any of the Constituent antigens. For example, if the minimum recommended interval between two doses of MMR is 4 weeks and two doses of varicella is 12 weeks, minimum interval between two doses of MMRV should not be less than 12 weeks.

c) Contraindication to one of the component antigen must be considered as contraindication for all combination vaccines containing that antigen. For example, contraindication for DPT e.g. anaphylaxis is a contraindication for all DPT containing combination vaccines.

d) In most of the currently available combination vaccines, component antigens are mixed at the level of manufacturer and no attempt should be made to mix them at the time of use indigenously, unless specifically licensed. e.g. mixing Pentavalent vaccine with IPV to make a hexavalent vaccine before administration is not advisable.

Frequently Asked Questions (FAQs)

1. **Why are live vaccines more immunogenic than inactivated vaccines?**

   Live vaccines are more immunogenic as – a) these vaccines replicate at the site to provide sustained supply of antigen, and b) Most attenuated pathogens still supply both B and T epitopes and consequently both humoral and cell-mediated responses are mounted, for long-lasting protection.

2. **Then, Why do some live vaccines need multiple doses?**

   Live vaccines are highly immunogenic and first dose usually provides enough protection. However, additional dose/s are *insurance* doses to ensure seroconversion of all recipients e.g. seroconversion rate after first dose on Measles vaccine is 95-98% and nearly 100% after two doses.

3. **Whether varicella vaccine can be given in private practice after a week of MR vaccine received by the child at a government hospital under NIS?**

   No. Both MR and varicella vaccines are live vaccines. Two or more live vaccines have to be given either on the same day or at least after 28 days interval as developing immune response (e.g. cytokines and interferon), to the first inoculation might affect the response to subsequent vaccine. This rule does not apply to live oral vaccines, which can be given together with other live or inactivated vaccines at any time interval.

4. **Is it also necessary to maintain 28 days interval between two inactivated, toxoid or subunit vaccines?**

   Unlike live vaccines, response to inactivated antigens is

usually not affected by circulating antibodies and hence, these vaccines can be given at any time interval with other vaccines or natural infections.

However, an exception is PCV-13 and MCV (Menectra®) in a high-risk case, which should be given only after 28 days of interval – PCV followed by Menectra®. Exception is not applicable to another brand of MCV - Menveo®.

5. **Why more than two doses of Polysaccharide vaccines are generally not recommended?**

Revaccination with polysaccharide vaccines might induce lower antibody responses than the first dose, a phenomenon termed as *immunological hyporesponsiveness*. Hence, more than two doses are generally not recommended.

6. **Whether a person allergic to neomycin can be given MMR or IPV vaccine?**

Neomycin is used as to prevent bacterial contamination of cultures during the manufacturing phase of some vaccines e.g. MMR, IPV etc. and very minute traces (<25 µg) may be left behind in finished products. Persons with known history of allergy to neomycin may be given these vaccines but should be closely observed after vaccination for any allergic reaction.

7. **What is the significance of presence of Thiomersal in a vaccine?**

Thiomersal is a commonly used preservative in many vaccines, specially multidose vials and may be responsible for some of the minor local reactions at injection site. Major concern with its use in vaccines is the possibility of neurological toxicity due to presence of ethyl mercury in it and some earlier reports linked it with autism in children. Some countries have mandated the use of thiomersal-free vaccines in their programs. However the Global Advisory Committee on Vaccine Safety did not find any conclusive evidence of association between thiomersal containing vaccines and autism or other neurological events. Recommendations for the removal of thiomersal in some countries are mainly driven by public perception of risk and not by any scientific evidence.

8. What are the advantages and disadvantages of adjuvants in a vaccine

Adjuvants improve the immunogenicity of a vaccine by many mechanisms e.g. a) slow but sustained release of antigens from injection site, b) attracting immune cells to enhance antigen uptake and presentation, c) modulation of The responses with induction of cytokines and chemokines, and d) promoting antigen transport to draining lymph nodes.

However, presence of an adjuvant may increase the incidence of local side-effects of a vaccine e.g. sterile abscess, nodules, granuloma or contact hypersensitivity.

References

1. Agrawal M. Immunization. *In*: Agrawal M. Textbook of Pediatrics. 2nd ed. New Delhi: CBS Publishers, 2017; pp 132-150.
2. American Academy of Pediatrics Vaccine Ingredients. *In*: Red Book® 2021-2024 Report of the Committee on Infectious Diseases. Kimberlin Et al (Eds), 32nd Edition, 2021; pg 17-19.
3. Global Alliance for Vaccines and Immunizations: Available from: https://www.gavi.org/vaccineswork/what-ingredients-go-vaccine?gclid=CjwKCAjw r56IBhAvEiwA1fuqGpYnmXk2zRU4fl-lgfrbqH3DP3DPIb7VQmsgawPkcfXW PEVDaOw8phoCxHIQAvD_BwE (Accessed July 6th, 2021).
4. Rathi N. Combination Vaccines In: Vashishtha V et al. FAQs on Vaccines and immunization practices. 2nd Edition. New Delhi, Jaypee Brothers 2015; pp 323-330.
5. Kumar P. Newer adjuvants. *In*: Vashishtha V et al. FAQs on Vaccines and immunization practices. 2nd Edition. .New Delhi, Jaypee Brothers 2015; pp 391-407.

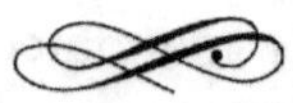

Immunogenicity & Efficacy of Vaccines

Success of a vaccine is generally denoted in terms of the *Immunogenicity* and the *Protective Efficacy*. These two terms, though often used interchangeably, have different connotations. Another term, *Protective effectiveness*, further adds to this confusion. This chapter deals with various indicators used to denote efficacy of a vaccine and factors which can affect it.

3.1: IMMUNOGENICITY

Immunogenicity of a vaccine is the *ability to induce disease-specific antibodies* after administration, which is commonly referred by two terms -

a) *Seroconversion rate i.e.* percentage of vaccines who achieve the pre-defined antibody titer after a defined period of vaccination, which is considered as protective. This protective threshold of antibodies is denoted as *"Correlate of protection"*. These correlates for vaccines predominantly acting through humoral immunity are relatively better defined and standardized (Table 3.1) then for those vaccines which predominantly act through cellular immunity.

Seroconversion rate is a qualitative parameter that dichotomously differentiates immunized persons as seroconverted or not seroconverted. However, all seroconverted cases may not essentially be protected against the disease on exposure. Conversely, many cases without adequate seroconversion may still be protected due to other reasons, discussed later.

Seroconversion rates for common vaccines after all recommended doses are provided in Table 3.1. However

Table 3.1: Correlates of protection[4], Seroconversion rates & Protective efficacy of Vaccines

Vaccine	Correlates of protection	Seroconversion rate*	Protective efficacy*
BCG	–	–	~60%[#]
Hepatitis B	≥ 10 mIU/ml	>95-99%	~100%
Diphtheria	≥ 0.1 IU/ml	>95%	>95%
Tetanus	≥ 0.01 IU/ml	~100%	>95%
Petusis (wP)	MICB	75-80%	75-80%
Petusis (aP)	≥ 5 U Elisa toxin	75-80%	75-80%
H. influenza B	≥ 0.15 µg/ml	–	95-100%
Polio (OPV)	–	65-70%	~100%
Polio (IPV)	–	~100%	~100%
Rotavirus	NA (IgA)	–	50-60% (in India)[#]
Pneumococcal (Conjugate)	≥ 0.35 µg/ml	80% for serotypes	~100%
Measles	≥ 120 mIU/ml	80-95%	>95%
Mumps	–	>90%	78-85%
Rubella	≥ 10 mIU/ml	>99%	>99%
JE	≥ 1:10 (N'Ab)	–	>80%
Influenza (IIV)	≥ 1:40 (HAI)		~60%
HAV	≥ 20 mI U/ml	90-95%	95-100%
TPSV	≥ 1 µg/ml anti-vi	>90%	55-70% for 2-3 yrs
TCV	≥ 1 µg/ml anti-vi	>98%	>98%
Varicella	≥5 IU/ml gp-ELISA	>75-85%	70-75% (>99% for severe disease)
MCV	≥ 1:4 N'Ab	96-100%	85-90%
HPV	NA	95-99%	~99% for CIN 2/3
Yellow fever	–	>99%	>99%

MICB: Murine intracerebral challenge test, **N'Ab:** Neutralizing Antibodies, **HAI:** Hemagglutination antibodies
* After all recommended doses
# Higher for severe disease

seroconversion rate is usually highest within 4-8 weeks of vaccination and tends to decline over time in absence of further exposures, as antibody titers in some cases decline and drop below the protective threshold.

b) *Geometric mean titer (GMT)* is a quantitative parameter to denote average of the *antibody* titers achieved by a group of immunized subjects, calculated by multiplying all values and taking the nth root of this number.

Higher GMT titers generally indicate stronger immune response with longer persistence above the protective threshold. However, GMT may also hide the number of non-responders in the group by averaging of the data.

Immunogenicity depends on characteristics of the - a) vaccine e.g. type of antigen, Presence of adjuvant, dose, route and site of administration, timing of doses etc. as well as of the - b) host e.g. Age, immunological status, co-morbidities etc. (Sec 3.3).

In brief, Immunogenicity of a vaccine is largely assessed in laboratories in terms of antibodies titers, which may or may not be protective in real life.

3.2: PROTECTIVE EFFICACY & EFFECTIVENESS

Clinical efficacy of a vaccine to reduce the risk of contracting disease on exposure is generally denoted by two terms – *Protective efficacy* and *Protective effectiveness*.

Protective efficacy of a vaccine refers to *reduction in the risk of disease on exposure due to a vaccine under trial conditions.* It is assessed in phase III studies by vaccinating only one group of subjects and comparing the incidence of disease in vaccinated group with another group of unvaccinated subjects in follow-up period.

Protective Efficacy is calculated as follows -

Vaccine Efficacy = Attack rate in unvaccinated population - Attack rate in vaccinated population / Attack rate in unvaccinated population x 100

Protective efficacy of a vaccine does not necessarily corresponds with seroconversion rate as antibody titers below protective thresholds may still be protective due to other reasons such as development of immune-memory or T cell immunity. Protective Efficacy of common vaccines after all recommended doses are provided in Table 1.

Protective Effectiveness is another term used in context of vaccine efficacy which denotes *"the extent to which a vaccine provides beneficial result* i.e. reduces the incidence of disease in general population in real-life conditions.

Protective effectiveness of a vaccine may exceed the protective efficacy due to phenomena like Contact immunity, Herd immunity and Herd effect, discussed below.

Contact immunity refers to the *"indirect immunization of non-vaccinated individuals through the vaccine-virus shed in stools or nasal secretions of an individual vaccinated with a live vaccine"* For example, OPV provides efficient contact immunity and Rotavirus vaccine is also expected to do so, though evidence is lacking.

Herd effect refers to *"Reduction of infection or disease in the unimmunized population as a result of the immunizing a proportion of the population"* The chain of transmission of a contagious infection is likely to be disrupted when a large number of population becomes immune due to immunization. Greater is the proportion of individuals who are resistant, smaller is the probability that a susceptible individual will come into contact with an infectious individual and get infection. Herd effect is largely seen with vaccines against diseases with direct human-to-human transmission e.g. PCV and HIB vaccines and not with others e.g. Tetanus in which only the vaccinated individuals are protected from disease. Herd effect may be the only protection to individuals who cannot be immunized due to medical reasons e.g. Immunocompromized states.

Herd effect can be measured by quantifying the *decline in incidence of infection in unvaccinated population* on follow up epidemiological studies after the inclusion of a vaccine in wide spread immunization program or intervention.However, reduction in the incidence of disease may also be due to other measures taken to prevent the spread of infection e.g. improvement in hygiene etc, which reduce the probability of transmission of infection in the community. It is determined by herd immunity as well as the force of transmission of the corresponding infection.

Herd protection is another commonly used term referring to *"the protection offered to the unimmunized individuals that remain protected in a herd by virtue of Herd-effect rendered by immunized individuals"* These individuals, if move out of that herd or population, will be at risk again due to withdrawal of herd protection.

3.3: DETERMINANTS OF IMMUNOGENECITY & EFFICACY

Efficacy of a vaccine depends on many known and hitherto unknown factors, including those related to the vaccine formulation, dosage schedule and recipient characteristics, as follows –

1. **Type of the Antigen:** Live vaccines are generally superior to Inactivated or conjugated vaccines, which are in turn better than polysaccharide vaccines, in terms of adequate and sustained immune response. *Live vaccines* are highly immunogenic due to sustained supply of antigen by endogenous replication of inoculated organism and provide robust and long-lasting immunity. On the other

hand, *inactivated vaccines* carry limited antigenic load per dose and hence, are poorly immunogenic with first dose and need multiple doses to achieve adequately protective titers.

Polysaccharide vaccines produce T-cell independent response, mainly of IgM class with no production of memory B cells and no anamnestic response on re-exposure. Hence, these vaccines are very poorly immunogenic, being gradually replaced by conjugate vaccines.

Conjugated vaccines are polysaccharide vaccines conjugated with another antigen e.g. toxoid to behave like inactivated T-cell dependent vaccines. Initial response to these vaccines is similar to that for polysaccharide vaccines but with development of memory B cells and potent anamnestic response of re-exposure. These vaccines too, like inactivated vaccines, require multiple doses for adequate and sustained immune response.

2. **Quantitative dose of Antigen:** As a general rule, higher dose of the antigen in a vaccine increases the immunogenicity. Immunocompromized children are often recommended double-dose of the HBV vaccine for adequate immune response. However, higher doses also increase the risk of side effects and increasing the antigenic dose beyond a limit is not recommended.

3. **Presence of Adjuvants:** Adjuvants are pharmacological substances added in some of the inactivated and subunit vaccines to improve their immunogenicity by– a) slow but sustained modulation of antigen delivery (depot effect), b) modulation of The responses to increase cytokine production, and c) stimulation of dendritic cell maturation.

4. **Number of Doses:** Increasing the number of doses naturally increases immunogenicity and efficacy of a vaccine, specially in cases of inactivated vaccines. Immunocompromized child are often advised to take

additional dose/s of these vaccines. While one dose is generally enough for most of live vaccines, additional dose are frequently advised to ensure seroconversion of all recipients For example, seroconversion rate after first dose on measles is 95-98% and nearly 100% after two doses.

5. **Time-interval between Doses:** Appropriate time-spacing between the priming and subsequent doses of the inactivated vaccines is essential to achieve best immunological results. Since, maturation of B cells in germinal centers and formation of memory B cells take at least 4–6 months a 0,2,6 mo schedule is generally considered as most immunogenic for non-replicating vaccines. However, need to complete the immunization series as early as possible has necessitated use of one-month interval between doses of inactivated vaccines, which is less appropriate but acceptable option. However, minimal interval of 4 months between the last primary dose and booster dose is necessary to ensure adequate pool of memory B cells before the booster.

6. **Time-interval between different Vaccines:** When two different live vaccines diseases are given at an interval of less than one month, parallel immune responses may affect the uptake of later vaccine. Hence, two live vaccines should be given either on the same day or at least with one month interval. Immune response to inactivated vaccines is not affected in this manner, which can be given at any time interval.

7. **Route of administration** of a vaccine also determines the strength and nature of immune response. Intradermal vaccination of some vaccines can induce antibody responses comparable to intramuscular or subcutaneous route with lesser dose of antigen, though more difficult to deliver precisely. Mucosal administration (intranasal or oral) of some vaccines stimulates higher levels of mucosal IgA

antibodies to inhibit disease transmission with greater effectiveness than parenteral administration.

8. **Age of the vaccination:** Since vaccine preventable diseases generally affect young children, immunization schedules aim to protect them at earliest possible age, before the risk of exposure. However, two important factors negatively affect immune responses during young age - Maternal antibodies and immaturity of immune system.

Presence of maternal antibodies in first 3–6 months of life interferes with successful uptake of vaccines due to rapid elimination of the administered antigen. Inhibitory influence of pre-existing antibodies is more marked on live vaccines and hence, live viral vaccines e.g. Measles and Varicella are not recommended before 6 months of age. However maternal antibodies do not interfere with T-cell response or local immunity and vaccines which predominantly produce cellular or local immunity e.g. BCG or OPV respectively, or for which maternal antibodies are generally absent or non-interfering e.g. HBV, may be given at birth.

Physiologically immature immune system in first 2-3 month of life with fewer antigenic processing sites e.g. follicular dendritic cells and germinal centers, lower Immunoglobulin production and poor-T-helper cell response prevents satisfactory immune response to vaccines in early infancy. However, due to the compulsion of protecting the child as early as possible and for operational reasons, six week is regarded as the lowest age limit to begin primary doses. Limitations of young age immunization can be overcome to some extent, by increasing the number of doses or use of boosters at a later age. In older children, lesser number of doses are required to achieve comparable immunogenicity. Note that polysaccharide vaccines are not adequately immunogenic before 2 years of age and hence, used only in older children.

9. ***Immunocompetence of the recipient:*** Vaccination in preterms, malnourished and Immunocompromized children may not produce adequate immune response due to relative immune-incompetence. Although live attenuated vaccines may theoretically produce the disease in these cases, such complications are extremely rare and should not preclude the use of live vaccine immunization, except in moderate to severe immunodeficiency states as discussed in chapter 27. Cell mediated immunity may be affected in severe malnutrition, leading to poor response to BCG and other vaccines with cellular immunity.

10. ***Genetic factors in recipients:*** Immunological responses to same vaccine might differ between individuals due to genetic variability of major histocompatibility complex molecules (HLA-A2), largely due to differences in T cell responses. Gene polymorphisms in molecules critical for B and T cell activation/differentiation are also likely to affect antibody responses. Deficiencies in the terminal components of complement and properdin also result in impaired immune response.

11. **Presence of Pre-formed antibodies or inhibitory antimicrobials:** Presence of passive antibodies following administration of immunoglobulins interferes with development of adequate immune response by rapid elimination of vaccine-antigen and should be avoided. However, as the protective effect of vaccines may take many weeks to appear, it is sometimes necessary to give Immunoglobulin and vaccines together, specially for post-exposure prophylaxis e.g. in Rabies, Tetanus and Hepatitis B.

12. **Contact immunity and Herd effect:** Many vaccines benefit even the unvaccinated population, though various mechanisms i.e. Contact immunity and Herd Effect, discussed earlier. In such cases, the protective effectiveness of the vaccine might be higher than the expected due to these phenomena.

Frequently Asked Questions (FAQs)

1. Which is a better term to express the benefits of vaccines – Seroconversion rate or Protective efficacy?

Protective efficacy is a better term than the seroconversion rate for clinicians as it reflects to actual benefit of the vaccine i.e. reduction in the risk of disease on exposure. It is usually higher than the seroconversion rate as antibody titers may drop below protective thresholds over time but vaccine may still be protective due to its ability to induce immune-memory and produce strong anamnestic response on re-exposure or stimulation of cellular immunity. *Note:* Since T-cell independent polysaccharide vaccines e.g. PSPV, MPSV and TPSV do not produce immunological memory, seroconversion rate and protective efficacy is usually comparable for them.

2. How does the vaccination of a child might benefit other contacts as well?

When a live vaccine is administered via mucosal route (oral/ Intranasal) e.g. OPV or Influenza (Live), virus is shed in stools or nasal secretions, leading to indirect immunization of unvaccinated contacts. *(Contact immunity).*

Note: Same phenomena may also be harmful, as live vaccines given to the contact of immunocompromised person can spread the infection to him and cause disease e.g. VAPP/VDPV or influenza.

3. Why does the expanding coverage of immunization with some vaccines reduce incidence of disease even in unimmunized population?

Expanding coverage of a vaccine with increasing proportion of resistant population reduces the probability of a susceptible individual coming in contact of an infectious person, thus breaking the chain of transmission. *(Herd effect).* Herd effect is largely seen with vaccines against diseases with direct human-to-human transmission e.g. PCV and HIB vaccines and not with others e.g. Tetanus in which only the vaccinated individuals are protected from disease. Herd effect may be the only protection to individuals who cannot be immunized due to medical reasons e.g. Immunocompromized states.

4. *Whether Herd immunity and Herd effect are synonymous?*

   No. the term *Herd effect* refers to *"Reduction of disease in the unimmunized population due to immunizing a proportion of the population"*, as these immunized subjects disrupt the chain of transmission in a community, indirectly benefitting unimmunized population.

   However, the term *Herd immunity* refers to *"overall proportion of subjects with immunity in a population, achieved either by immunization or after natural exposure"*, discounting the indirect protection to unimmunized and un-exposed population.

5. **An American child, though unvaccinated for PCV, never contracted the disease while staying there, perhaps due to Herd effect. Whether he will also be protected, if moves to India?**

   No. The protection offered to the unimmunized individuals by virtue of herd effect (*Herd Protection*) is available only till they are the part of that herd as large number of immunized persons will not contract and transmit the disease to unimmunized subjects. However, once moved out of that herd, he will be at risk of infection again due to withdrawal of this herd protection. (PCV coverage is presently very low in India, though vaccine is being introduced gradually in NIS.

6. **What is a "Correlate of protection"?**

   The term *correlate of protection* denotes a measurable and standardized immunological marker induced in response to a vaccine, which is considered as protective (Table 3.1). These correlates are important to assess the immunogenicity of a vaccine and compare effect of different vaccines.

Specific *serum antibody titers* are most frequently used correlates of protection for vaccines inducing humoral immunity. These correlates may be directly protective e.g. Anti-HBSag titers following HBV vaccination, or surrogate markers e.g. gpElisa units for varicella or IgA levels for Rotavirus vaccine. Measurement of correlates for cellular components is difficult and diseases like pertussis and HPV have no established correlates.

References

1. Pemde H. Elementary Epidemiology *In:* IAP Guidebook on Immunization 2018-19 - Advisory Committee on Vaccines and Immunization Practices, Indian Academy of Pediatrics, 3rd Edition, New Delhi, Jaypee Brothers 2020; pp 28-34.
2. Vashishtha VM et al. Elementary Epidemiology in vaccination *In:* Vashishtha V et al. FAQs on Vaccines and immunization practices. 2nd Edition. .New Delhi, Jaypee brothers 2015; pp 24-31.
3. Weinberg GA et al. Vaccine epidemiology: Efficacy, effectiveness and the translational research roadmap. J Infect Dis. 2010;201:1607-10.
4. Plotkin SA. Correlates of Vaccine protection. Clinical and Vaccine immunology. 2010;17 (7): 1055–1065.
5. Khanna S et al. Epidemiology in relation to Vaccinology. *In:* IAP Textbook of Vaccines. Vashishtha VM et al (Editors). 1st edition, New Delhi, Jaypee Brothers 2014; pp 25-36.
6. Yash Paul. Herd Immunity and Herd Protection: Benefits and Harms to Community by Vaccines. *In:* IAP Textbook of Vaccines. Vashishtha VM et al (Editors). 1st edition, New Delhi, Jaypee Brothers 2014; pp 74-78.

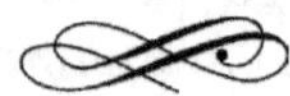

Storage, Transport & Handling of Vaccines

Vaccines, being biological agents, are likely to lose their potency when exposed to the detrimental environmental conditions e.g. heat and light. Efficient vaccine storage and handling is a key component of immunization programs.

Vaccines stored or transported at temperatures other than recommended range may become less effective, ineffective or even risky to use. It is often difficult to reliably assess the potency of a vaccine at the delivery point and the use of sub-optimal vaccine products can lead to immunization failures, loss of public confidence in immunization programs and wastage of resources. Inappropriate vaccine handling can occur at the level of manufacture, transport, storage or administration and studies have shown that 17-37% health-care providers expose vaccines to improper storage conditions.

Storage/Transport requirements: Each vaccine has own storage/transport requirements, generally as follows –

- *Heat-sensitive vaccines:* Live vaccines are more susceptible to heat, maximum being Varicella followed in descending order of sensitivity by OPV, MR/MMR, BCG, Yellow fever and some RV vaccines. However, these vaccines are relatively *freeze-tolerant* and can be used if frozen, though repeated freezing-thawing should be avoided

- *Freeze-sensitive vaccines:* Vaccines containing aluminium adjuvants e.g. Tetanus containing vaccines, HBV, HAV, HPV and PCV as well as some others e.g. IPV, IIV, MCV/MPSV, TCV/TPSV, Hib etc are cold-sensitive and deteriorate on thawing, if frozen. These vaccines should be discarded, if frozen accidentally.

- *Light-sensitive vaccines:* BCG, MR/MMR, Varicella, HPV and DTaP/Tdap vaccines are light sensitive and should not be exposed to sunlight or strong fluorescent lights. These vaccines are usually supplied in dark vials and should be stored in dark place.

Desired temperature zone for storage and transport of most vaccines is 2–8°C though highly heat-sensitive vaccines e.g. OPV, need to be stored or transported at -15 to -25°C for long-term storage from central depot to district depots level.

Cold Chain is an operational term to define *a system of transporting and storing the vaccines at recommended temperatures from the manufacturers' level till the point of administration.*

Essential components of cold chain include:

a. **Equipment** i.e. use of appropriate equipment to maintain the desired temperature during transport, storage and immunization sessions;

b. **Personal** i.e. appropriate training of the persons involved in handling of vaccines at all points i.e. storage, transport, distribution and delivery.

c. **Procedure** i.e. standard operating protocol and quick transport facilities to decrease the risk of exposure to high temperatures,

d. **Surveillance** i.e. Continuous as well as periodic *surveillance* for efficacy of cold chain maintenance.

4.1: COLD-CHAIN EQUIPMENTS

Cold-chain Equipments to maintain adequate cold chain system differ according to the purpose i.e. storage *vs* transfer, volume of vaccines which need to be stored/transported and logistics i.e. electricity supply. Equipments used in large-volume public sector are often difficult to use in private facilities. Table 1 summarizes common cold-chain storage equipments used at different centers.

Some important storage or transport cold-chain equipments are as follows –

Walk-in Coolers/Freezers (WIC/WIF) are large vaccine storage facilities, used at central or regional vaccine depots for bulk storage of vaccines. WIC/WIF are made up of insulated panels, maintain temperatures at 2-8°C (WIC) or -15 to -25°C (WIF) and have advanced continuous temperature monitoring systems with warning alarms (**Fig. 4.1**). WIF are used for bulk storage of OPV vaccine along with preparation and storage of ice-packs while WIC are used for storage of other vaccines. These WIC/WIF are generally used to store 3 months' supply of vaccines along with additional 25% buffer stock.

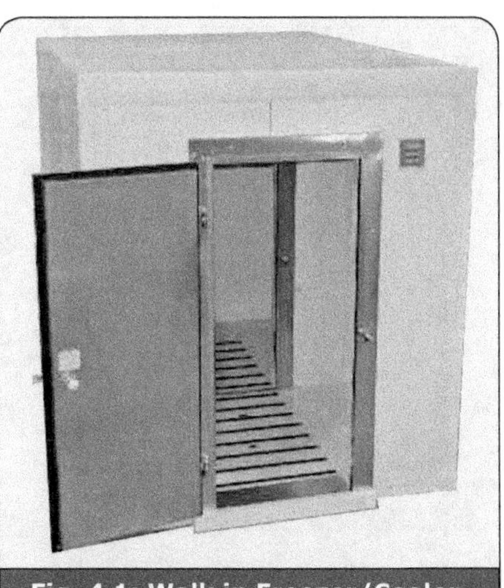

Fig. 4.1: Walk in Freezer/Cooler.

Deep Freezers (DF) are usually top-open refrigeration systems, used to store OPV at the district level at -18 to -20°C along with preparation and storage of ice-packs.

Ice-lined Refrigerator (ILR) is a top-open refrigerator with a lining of ice packs inside the walls to maintain the temperature within the safe range (2–8°C), even if the electricity fails. ILRs are used to store all vaccines at primary health centers where power supply is often erratic. ILR can keep vaccines safe for 24 hours even with as little as 8-hour of continuous electricity supply.

ILR has two sections—the top basket and the bottom. While heat-sensitive vaccines e.g. OPV, MR/MMR, BCG, RV etc must be stored at the bottom which is the coolest part, freeze-sensitive vaccines should be stored in the basket to avoid freezing, including those returned under open vial policy. ILRs should not be used to store anything other than vaccines, including drugs and expired date vaccines. Top-open lid minimizes the loss of cold air while opening the door, though it should not be opened frequently (**Fig. 4.2**).

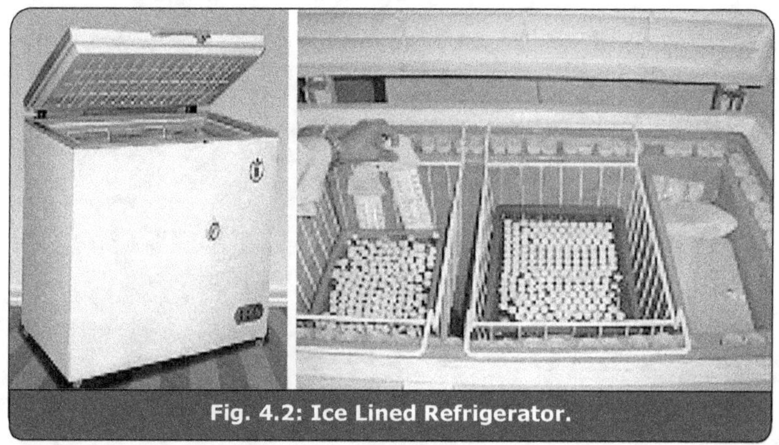

Fig. 4.2: Ice Lined Refrigerator.

Vaccine van is an insulated van used for bulk transport of vaccines from central or regional depots to district centers. Vaccines should be transported only in cold boxes, which should be loaded in the vaccine van immediately after packing. At destination, these boxes must be unloaded as early as possible and vaccines should be transferred to the ILR immediately.

Cold Boxes (Coolers) are large (20-25 Litre) or small (5-8 Litre) insulated boxes, used for transportation of vaccines to peripheral health centers. These boxes can also be used to store vaccines and frozen ice packs in case of power failures with hold-over time of 48-96 hours at 43°C. A dial thermometer is kept inside to record the temperature. Before placing vaccines in these boxes, fully frozen ice packs need to be placed at the bottom and sides of the box. The vials of DPT, DT, TT, HBV etc. should first be wrapped in plastic sheets or kept in cartons before keeping inside, to avoid freezing.

Vaccine carriers *or isothermic boxes* are small insulated boxes used to carry small amount of vaccines from refrigerator to the immunization site. In these carriers, a safe temperature of 2-8°C can be maintained for 6–8 hours (even upto 24 hours, if not opened frequently), using frozen ice packs lined on the side of the box. The vials of DPT, DT and TT should first be wrapped in plastic sheets before keeping inside, to avoid freezing (**Fig. 4.3**).

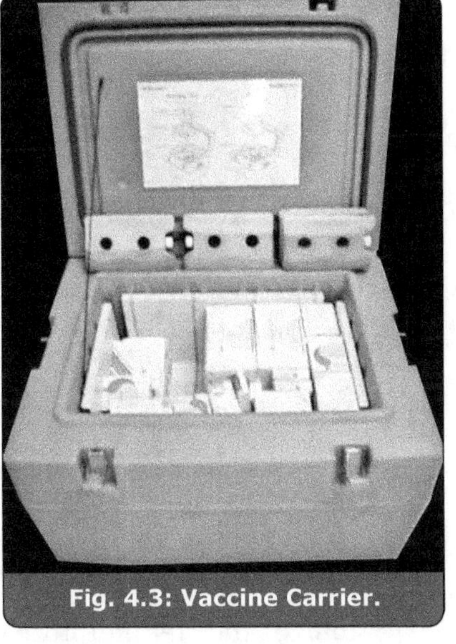

Fig. 4.3: Vaccine Carrier.

Domestic Refrigerator, though frequently used in private sector to store vaccines, is not ideal solution as it does not have accurate temperature controlling system with wild temperature fluctuations during frosting-defrosting cycles and door opening. However, it is an acceptable alternative in absence of other facilities provided –

a) It is frost-free, which have no heating cycles but have low-level warming cycles and hence provides more uniform temperatures than manual and cyclic defrost models.

b) It has separate external door for Freezer compartments, with automatic closure and tight seals.

c) It is accessible only to vaccination staff and is not used to store anything other than vaccines e.g. drugs, water etc.

d) Refrigerator compartment temperatures is maintained at 2-8°C and freezer compartment temperatures is maintained at or below 5°F. (−15°C).

Some important precautions for use of domestic refrigerator for vaccine storage are as follows (**Fig. 4.4**) -

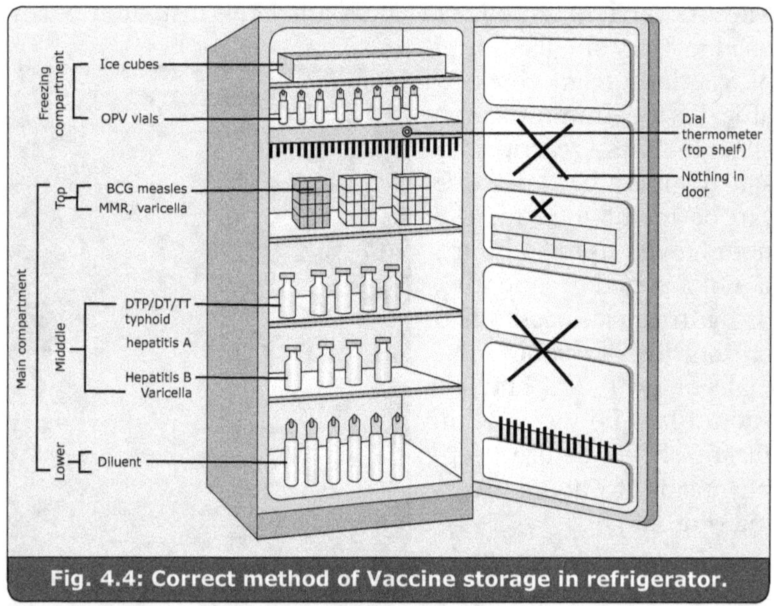

Fig. 4.4: Correct method of Vaccine storage in refrigerator.

- Stabilize the temperature of the refrigerator before stocking the vaccines:

- Place ice packs/gel packs in the refrigerator, below the bottom shelf, to increase the cooling mass and to stabilize temperature during warming cycles, door opening, short-time electricity failures and refrigerator malfunctions.

- Store vaccines in original packing and transparent labeled containers for easier identification and minimizes the door-open time.

- Do not store any vaccine in the freezer, chiller, door or basket. Store *freeze-tolerant vaccines in the top shelf, other freeze-sensitive vaccines on the middle shelf and diluents in the lower compartment* of refrigerator section. Ice packs can be kept in freezer. Never put freeze-sensitive vaccines in contact or close to evaporator plate of refrigerator.

- Do not overstock and overload refrigerator with vaccines.

Keep at least 4 cm space from the walls and containers to allow free air circulation.

- Do not store vaccines or diluents in the door shelves.

- Keep a thermometer in the upper shelf to monitor the temperature, preferably a digital one with memory record of minimum/maximum temperature and alarms.

- In case of power failure, use a backup generator facility. If not available, shift the vaccines to a cool box with ice packs if power failure lasts or expected to last for more than 4 hours and move to an pre-identified alternative storage facility, if necessary.

- Identify a dedicated person/staff, who should only be permitted to handle Vaccine refrigerator.

Purpose-built Refrigerator, built specifically for vaccine storage purpose, is used by hospitals, pharmacies, and larger general practices. These refrigerators provide more stable and even temperature at 2-8°C control along with monitoring and alarms.

Table 4.1: Common cold-chain equipment used under UIP at different Storage centers		
Site	**For OPV**	**For other vaccines**
CXentral & state Depots	Walk-In-Freezer (-15 to -25°C)	Walk-In-Cooler (2-8°C)
District centers	Deep Freezer (-15 to -25°C)	Ice-lined refrigerator (2-8°C)
Primary health center	Ice-lined refrigerator (2-8°C)	Ice-lined refrigerator (2-8°C)
Sub-centers	Cold boxes (2-8°C)	Cold boxes (2-8°C)
Immunization sites	Vaccine carrier (2-8°C)	Vaccine carrier (2-8°C)
Private Practice	Purpose built Refrigerator* (2-8°C)	Purpose built Refrigerator* (2-8°C)

Hold-over time (at 43°C): Deep freezer 2.5 hours, Ice-lined refrigerator 20 hours, Cold box 48-96 hours, Vaccine carrier 36 hours.
* Avoid domestic refrigerators

4.2: COLD-CHAIN MONITORING

Temperature monitoring is a critical component of cold chain to ensure that vaccines are stored and transported at recommended temperatures and involves use of - a) manual thermometers, (b) electronic data loggers and indicators and c) vaccine vial monitors. A break in the cold chain is indicated, if the temperature exceeds above 8°C or falls below 2°C in the WIC/ILR and above -15°C in the WIF/DF. Random vaccine samples are also collected from distribution and field sites for laboratory potency testing.

Dial thermometer, though used commonly, are often not accurate and indicate the temperature only at the time of reading. Temperature fluctuations outside the recommended range at other times are missed. If used, the temperature on dial thermometer must be read at least twice a day and plotted on a chart to show high/low excursions (**Fig. 4.5**).

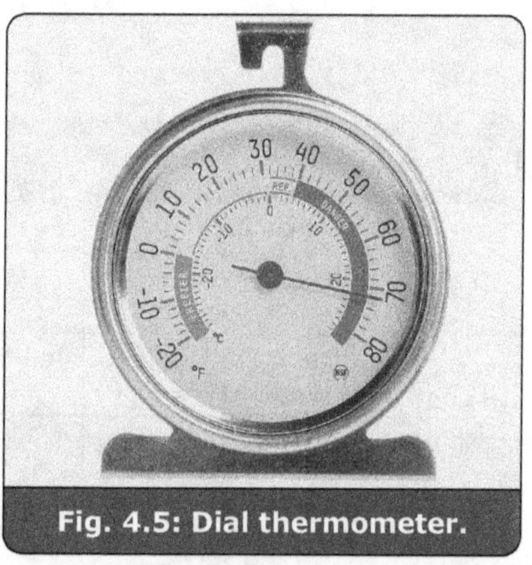

Fig. 4.5: Dial thermometer.

Alcohol stem thermometers are more sensitive and accurate than dial thermometers, which can record temperatures from -40°C to +50°C and can be used for ILRs or DFs.

Minimum/Maximum Thermometer are fluid-filled or digital devices to show the current temperature and the minimum and maximum temperatures achieved, indicating fluctuations outside the recommended range. Probe must be placed directly in contact with a vaccine vial or package and Thermometer must be reset regularly.

Data Loggers are miniature electronic systems for real-time temperature monitoring with digital display. These systems have multiple sensors, which can be placed at different locations of refrigerator (ILR) and can track a record of the temperatures at different sites over as long as 30 days to build up a "temperature map". Different sensors also help to identify problem-areas for temperature fluctuations in the storage equipment. These loggers also provide visual and audio alarms, even the SMS alerts, on significant temperature fluctuations.

Freeze indicator (Freeze-tag®) is an electronic device to monitor exposure of Freeze-sensitive vaccines (Penta, HBV, IPV etc) to freezing temperature, when placed along with these vaccines. On exposure of the indicator to a temperature below 0°C for more than 60 minutes, the LCD display will change from the "good" to the "alarm". and status "X". Vaccines should never be used without conducting the shake test when freeze tag shows the "X" mark. Freeze indicators can not be used once changed to alarm status and must be discarded (**Fig. 4.6**).

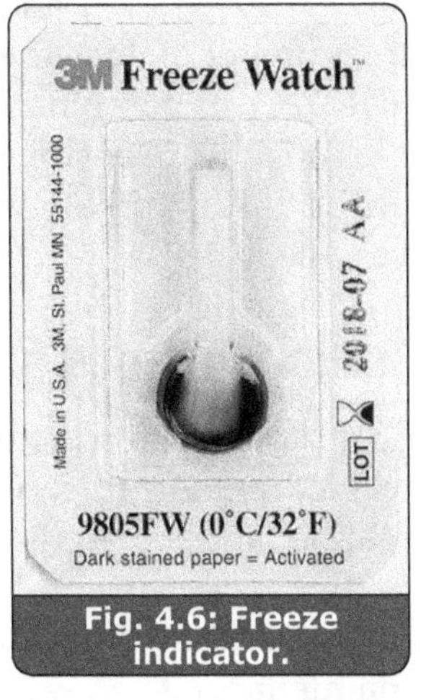

Fig. 4.6: Freeze indicator.

Vaccine Vial Monitor is a sticker fixed over the heat-sensitive vaccine vials to identify whether the vaccine has been damaged by exposure to heat and should not be used. It includes a lighter square made of a heat-sensitive material inside a darker circle (**Fig. 4.7**). On exposure to higher ambient temperatures, the color of the square darkens irreversibly. *If the color of square is darker or matching the outer circle, vaccine is probably not potent and should be discarded.*

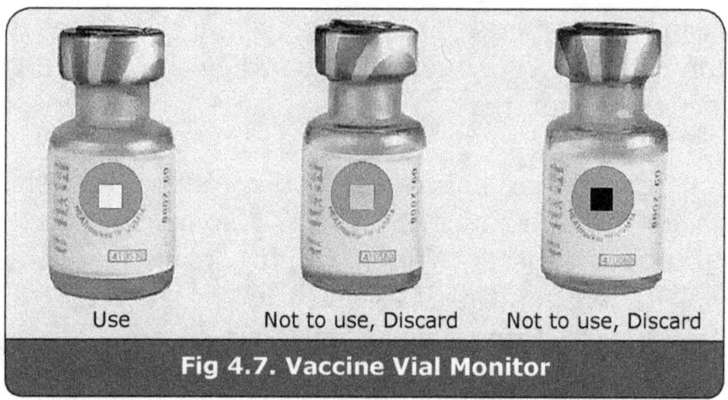

Fig 4.7. Vaccine Vial Monitor

VVM is not a substitute of expiry date and vaccine may also degrade due to other factors e.g. light exposure, which is not indicated by VVM.

VVMs are unique to each vaccine and are of four types - VVM 30, VVM 14, VVM 7 and VVM 2, with number corresponding to the number of days the vaccine remains potent with exposure at +37°C. In combination vaccines, the VVM corresponds to the most heat-sensitive component of the vaccines, e.g. VVM on DPT vial corresponds to the Pertussis component of the vaccine.

4.3: COLD-CHAIN PROTOCOLS (SOPS)

Each vaccination clinic should have a designated and trained person to coordinate the vaccine supply, cold-chain maintenance, handling and distribution activities along with a back-up staff. In addition, all staff must be trained to understand the importance and basic principles of cold chain maintenance.

It is always better to have written protocol for– a) vaccine inventory and procurement, b) cold-chain maintenance including emergency plan, and c) handling including post-use disposal or re-use (Open vial policy).

Some important components of such protocols are as follows –

- Keep the vaccine procurement *need-based* as per expected requirement during the procurement cycle plus another 25% for back-up, to avoid unnecessary storage problems.

- Maintain a vaccine inventory log including quantity, batch number, expiry date and date of procurement.

- Ensure that the storage facility is available and working at the time of expected delivery, before ordering the procurement.

- On arrival, transfer the vaccines immediately to storage equipment at recommended temperatures. Rotate the stock so vaccine and diluent with the shortest expiry date is used first.

- Keep a map of vaccine locations outside of the refrigerator door so that staff can go "straight" to the vaccine when the door is opened.

- Inspect the storage unit regularly to ensure that vaccines and thermometers are placed appropriately within the unit.

- Identify and designate an alternate site for vaccine storage/ shifting in case of equipment/power failure at primary site beyond the recommended time. Adequate Packing material (cold box, gel packs etc) must be available to shift the vaccines, if required.

- Remove expired or potentially compromised vaccines (and diluents) from the storage unit immediately and dispose off as early as possible.

- Have a written policy for storage, emergency transport and handling of vaccines with necessary contact numbers.

Frequently Asked Questions (FAQs)

1. **What is hold-over time?**

   Hold-over time is the duration for which a cold-chain equipment can maintain the temperature within its recommended range, in case of equipment/power failure. For example, Hold-over time for ILR is 20 hours at 43°C and it means that at an ambience temperature of 43°C, ILR can maintain inside cabinet temperature <8°C for minimum 20 hours. Hold-over time is adversely affected by high ambient temperature, frequent opening of lids, overloading quantity of vaccines and melted/partially frozen ice packs used in lining.

Hold-over time at 43°C for various equipments is – Deep freezer (2.5 hours), Ice line refrigerator (20 hours), Cold box (48-96 hours) and Vaccine carrier (36 hours).

2.   **What is Open-vial policy?**

Open-vial policy has been implemented since 2017, to permit the reuse of partially used multi-dose vials in subsequent sessions up to 28 days, subject to certain conditions. This policy helps to reduce the wastage and is applicable only for Pentavalent vaccine, OPV, HBV, PCV and IPV. It is not applicable for BCG, MR, Rotavirus and Japanese encephalitis vaccines. To use a vaccine under Open vial policy, following conditions must be fulfilled –

- Vial is within the expiry date and the VVM has not reached the discard point,

- Label is legible and date and time of previous use is written on vial,

- Vial was stored in appropriate cold-chain conditions during transportation and use,

- Vial septum was not submerged in water or contaminated in any way,

- Vial is not frozen, does not contain foreign body or has no cracks/leaks,

- Proper aseptic technique was used to withdraw vaccine doses,

- Vial was not involved in any AEFI event.

3. **Whether an acceptable VVM reading indicates that the vaccine is potent?**

    Not necessarily. VVM indicates that vaccine has not been damaged due to heat exposure beyond the permissible limits. VVM is not a substitute of expiry date and vaccine may also degrade due to other factors e.g. light exposure.

4. **How should diluents be stored in cold chain system?**

    Diluents should be stored, preferably in zip-lock packs, at the last cold chain point of the ILR. In case of space constraint, diluents may also be stored outside but must be kept in cold chain (2-8°C) at least 24 hours before use to ensure identical temperature of vaccine and diluents. Use of high temperature diluents may affect viability of live organisms in the vaccine (*Thermal shock*). Diluents and droppers of the vaccines must be essentially carried in the vaccine carrier during transport to vaccination site.

5. **What is *conditioning* of ice packs?**

    Ice packs are plastic containers filled with water and hard frozen in the deep freezer at about -20°C. They need to be kept at room temperature for some time to un-freeze to prevent damage to freeze-sensitive vaccines during transportation, if they come in direct contact with the frozen ice packs. This process is called *"conditioning"*. To condition, remove the frozen pack from deep freezer and place them on a flat surface. Shake one of the ice packs every few minutes. The ice is conditioned as soon as it begins to move about slightly inside its container.

6. **How can one check the potency of freeze-sensitive vaccines, if suspected frozen accidentally.**

    Freeze sensitive vaccines e.g. Penta, IPV, HBV etc. may lose their potency, if frozen, with higher risk of adverse events. e.g. sterile abscesses. Accidentally frozen vials of these vaccines must be discarded. However, if large number of vials are suspected (but not confirmed) to be frozen, ***Shake test*** can be used to check the status as follows –

- Take one of the suspected frozen vial and label it as *"Test vial"*.

- Take another vial of the same batch, which was stored properly, freeze it overnight at -20°C in the deep freezer, label it as *"Control vial"* and then thaw it without heating.

- Hold *Control vial* and the *Test vial* together and shake vigorosly for 10-15 seconds.

- Rest both vials side to side on a flat surface and observe for 30 min to compare for rate of sedimentation.

- If the sedimentation rate in the *Test vial* is slower than in the *Control vial*, the vaccine is not damaged. Discard the vaccines, if sedimentation rate is similar or faster in the test vial.

References

1. Shastri DD. Vaccine Storage and Handling *In:* IAP Guidebook on Immunization 2018-19 - Advisory Committee on Vaccines and Immunization Practices, Indian Academy of Pediatrics, 3rd Edition, New Delhi, Jaypee Brothers 2020; pp 50-68.
2. Shastri DD. Cold Chain and vaccine storage. *In:* Vashishtha V et al. FAQs on Vaccines and immunization practices. 2nd Edition. .New Delhi, Jaypee Brothers 2015; pp 76-84.
3. Vaccine Handling and storage, Red Book® 2021-2024 Report of the Committee on Infectious Diseases, American Academy of Pediatrics. Kimberlin *et al* (Eds), 32nd Edition, 2021; pg 19-25.
4. World Health organization. Immunization in practice: A practical guide for health staff – 2015 update. Module 2: The vaccine cold chain. pg 2(3) – 2(44).
5. Ministry of Health and Family welfare, Government of India. Managing the cold chain and Vaccine carrier. *In:* Immunization Handbook for health workers 2018; pp 67-78.

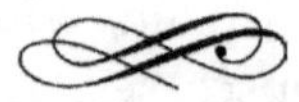

Immunization Schedules

Immunization schedules vary from country to country and need to be revised time to time, depending on the - a) Disease burden in the population, (b) Epidemiological characteristics, e.g. common age of infection, (c) Availability of safe and effective vaccine, (d) Economic feasibility and cost-effectiveness, and (e) logistic considerations.

An appropriate immunization schedule aims to -

- *Cover as many diseases of public health significance as possible* for which effective and safe vaccines are available. Some vaccines are used universally, while others are used only in selected at-risk population e.g. Japanese encephalitis.

- *Use vaccines with highest possible protective efficacy and safety*, within the available resources. Sometimes, a compromise is required on this aspect, e.g. countries with higher disease burden opt for a vaccine with higher protective efficacy (e.g. DTwP), compromising safety; while countries with lower disease burden are more concerned with safety issues, using vaccine with less side effects (e.g. DTaP).

- *Complete the Immunization before the risk of exposure begins, generally at the earliest possible age, as vaccine preventable diseases usually affect younger children.* HPV vaccine is given at or after 9 years of age when the risk of HPV infection begins to rise.

- *Schedule different vaccines at appropriate age* as per their immunogenicity profile e.g. Polysaccharide vaccines are not immunogenic in first two years of life and hence, used only in older children, if required.

- *Schedule the vaccines with appropriate number and interval of doses* to maximize protective efficacy. Usually Live vaccines require none or fewer number of doses than inactivated vaccines.

- *Provide Booster doses for the vaccines with shorter duration of protection* despite continued risk of exposure.

- *Minimize the number of pricks and visits* to complete planned immunization to avoid inconvenience to parents and *drop-outs*, using combination vaccines and clubbing multiple vaccinations at same visit.

Immunization schedule of a country is dynamic and needs periodic modifications to accommodate emerging diseases, changing epidemiology and newer vaccines. World Health Organization monitors vaccination schedules across the world including the coverage rates and issues broad guidelines to assist in decision-making.

Immunization Schedules In India

Currently, two schedules are followed in India – *National Immunization schedule (NIS)* for immunization of general population through public resources and *IAP Immunization schedule* recommended by Indian Academy of Pediatrics, for use in an individual child through private sector. Both schedules are often complementary and not contradictory.

Vaccines, currently used in India, may be broadly classified as:

a. *Essential vaccines included in NIS* (also termed as EPI vaccines), i.e. BCG, HBV, OPV, IPV, DPT, HIB, RV, PCV, MR and JE vaccines. Of these, DPT, HIB and HBV are given as a combination pentavalent vaccine for primary immunization; PCV vaccine has been recently introduced in NIS; and Japanese encephalitis vaccine is administered only in endemic districts. These vaccines are provided free-of charge by the Government.

b. ***Additional vaccines recommended by Indian Academy of Pediatrics (IAP)***, i.e. Influenza (< 5 years of age), MMR Typhoid, HAV, Varicella and HPV vaccines. These vaccines are advised over and above the EPI vaccines for use in private sector, subject to parental counseling and affordability. In some cases, IAP also recommends use of combination vaccines or a different vaccine for the same disease then that used in NIS (e.g. MMR instead of MR or Tdap instead of Td), due to various reasons.

c. ***Vaccines recommended in special circumstances only to high-risk children***, include vaccines for influenza (> 5 years), Meningococci, Rabies, Cholera and Yellow fever and some polysaccharides vaccines e.g. PPSV. These vaccines are used only in children at higher risk of disease, including post-exposure prophylaxis.

In addition, there are many *newer vaccines*, which are - a) either available in other countries but not yet approved in India, or b) Not yet approved for human usage, being under trials in various phases of development (Ch 25).

5.1: NATIONAL IMMUNIZATION SCHEDULE (NIS)

NIS in India currently aims to prevent *twelve* diseases in all children (and some in pregnant mothers), i.e. Tuberculosis, Diphtheria, Pertussis, Tetanus, Hepatitis B, H. influenzae B, Poliomyelitis, Rotavirus, Pneumococcal disease, Measles, Rubella and Japanese encephalitis, using ten vaccines, i.e. BCG, Pentavalent vaccine (DPT, HBV, Hib) OPV, IPV, RV, PCV, MR, JE , DPT and Td. JE vaccine is used only in selected endemic districts. Recently, PCV has been included for universal immunization and TT has been replaced by Td for use in pregnant mothers and older children at 10 and 16 years of age.

NIS has been adopted in all national child health programs and vaccines are provided by the government free of charge (**Table 5.1**).

Table 5.1: National Immunization Schedule of India

Vaccine	Due age	Max Age	Dose	Route	Site*
For Pregnant women					
Td1	Early in pregnancy	-	0.5 ml	IM	UA
Td2[2]	4 weeks later	-	0.5 ml	IM	UA
Td Booster[2]	If 2 doses received in last 3 years	-	0.5 ml	IM	UA
For Infants					
BCG	At birth	1 yr	0.05 ml[1]	ID	Lt UA
HBV (Birth dose)	At birth	24 hrs	0.5 ml	IM	Lt Thigh
OPV (Zero dose)	At birth	15 days	2 drops	PO	Oral
OPV 1, 2,3	6, 10, 14 wks	5 yrs	2 drops	PO	Oral
PentaV[3] 1, 2, 3	6, 10, 14 wks	1 yr	0.5 ml	IM	Lt Thigh
Fractional IPV	6, 14 weeks	1 yr	0.1 ml	ID	Rt UA
Rotavirus	6, 10, 14 wks	1 yr	5 drops	PO	Oral
PCV	6, 14 wks, 9 mo	1 yr	0.5 ml	IM	Rt Thigh
MR 1st dose	9-12 mo	5 yrs	0.5 ml	SC	Rt UA
J. Encephalitis-1[4]	9-12 mo	15 yrs	0.5 ml	SC	Lt UA
Vit A (1st dose)	9 mo	5 yrs	1 ml	PO	Oral
For Children					
DPT (B1)	16-24 mo	7 yrs	0.5 ml	IM	Lt Thigh
MR 2nd dose	16-24 mo	5 yrs	0.5 ml	SC	Rt UA
OPV (B)	16-24 mo	5 yrs	2 drops	PO	Oral
J. Encephalitis-2	16-24 mo	15 yrs	0.5 ml	SC	Lt UA
Vit A (2nd-9th dose)	16 mo > every 6 mo	5 yrs	2 ml	PO	Oral
DPT (B2)	5-6 yrs	7 Yrs	0.5 ml	IM	UA
Td	10 yrs & 16 yrs	16 Years	0.5 ml	IM	UA

Abbreviations: UA: Upper arm, Rt: Right, Lt: Left

[1] 0.1 ml after one month of age
[2] Preferably <36 weeks of pregnancy, but may be given later
[3] Combination DTwP, HBV and HIB vaccines
[4] In select endemic districts

5.2: IAP IMMUNIZATION SCHEDULE

NIS is the practical but not necessarily an ideal immunization schedule, as many useful vaccines have been left-out from universal immunization due to cost-considerations. Immunization schedule recommended by the Advisory Committee on Vaccines and Immunization Practices of IAP (ACVIP-IAP), henceforth referred as *IAP schedule,* aims to provide best possible immunization coverage to an individual child (**Table 5.2**).

Important differences between NIS and IAP guidelines are as follows:

- IAP recommends universal coverage to all healthy children for *six additional diseases– Mumps, Varicella, Hepatitis A, Typhoid, Influenza and HPV infections.*

- IAP recommends only *single dose of OPV at birth* instead of five doses in NIS. It recommends use of *IM-IPV for primary and booster doses* (along with OPV at birth) instead of combined OPV+fIPV primary schedule used in NIS followed by two booster doses of OPV. IM-IPV may be used as combination vaccine. If unaffording, child should be sent to government facility for primary schedule.

- IAP recommends use of *any - DTwP or DTaP* for primary and booster doses, instead of DTwP used in NIS. Further, a single dose of *Tdap* is recommended to all fully immunized children after 7 years of age instead of Td at 10 and 16 years. IAP also recommends Tdap instead of Td for immunization in pregnancy.

- IAP recommends that *last HBV dose should be administered not before 24 weeks of age and at least 16 weeks after first dose,* whichever is later, instead of 14 weeks of age in NIS.

- IAP recommends *four doses of PCV at 6,10,14 weeks with a booster at 15 months* instead of three doses at 6 weeks, 10 weeks and 9 months in NIS.

Table 5.2: IAP Immunization schedule		
Age	**Vaccine**	**Comments**
Birth	BCG OPV *(Zero dose)* HBV-1 *(Birth dose)*	BCG Before discharge OPV as soon as possible after birth HBV Within 24 hours of birth
6 weeks	DTwP/DTaP-1 IPV-1 HBV-2 HIB-1 RV-1 PCV-1	DTwP or DTaP may be administered in primary immunization IPV may be given as combination vaccine if unaffordable, child must be sent to government facility for primary immunization.
10 weeks	DTwP/DTaP-2 IPV-2 HBV-3 HIB-2 RV-2 PCV-2	RV1: Two-dose schedule Other RV vaccines: Three-dose schedule
14 weeks	DTwP/DTaP-3 IPV-3 HBV-4 HIB-3 RV-3 PCV-3	Additional 4th dose of HBV is safe, permitted in combination vaccines. RV3 is not indicated if RV1 vaccine (Rotarix) is used
6 months	Influenza (IIV)-1	Repeated every year in pre-monsoon season till 5 yr of age.
7 months	Influenza (IIV)-2	
6-9 months	TCV	Singe dose, No booster
9 months	MMR-1	
12 months	HAV-1	Only one dose for of Live attenuated vaccine
15 months	MMR-2 Varicella-1 PCV (B)	
16-18 months	DTwP/DTaP (B-1) IPV2 (B-1) HIB (B)	
18-19 months	HAV-2 Varicella-2	Only if inactivated HAV vaccine has been used
4-6 years	DTwP/DTaP (B-2) IPV2 (B-2) MMR-3	
10-12 years	Tdap	Even if has been administered earlier as DPT-B2
	HPV	Age 9-14 yrs: Two doses @ 0, 6 mo Age ≥15 yrs: Three doses @ 0, 1, 6 mo (HPV2) or 0, 2, 6 mo (HPV4)

Fig. 5.1: Indian Academy of pediatrics (ACVIP) recommended Immunization Schedule 2020-21

	Birth	6w	10w	14w	6m	7m	9m	12m	13m	15m	16-18m	18-24 m	2-3y	4-6y	9-14y	15-18y
BCG	BCG															
HBV	HBV$_1$ [a]	HBV$_2$	HBV$_3$	HBV$_4$ [b]												
Polio	OPV	IPV$_1$ [c]	IPV$_2$ [c]	IPV$_3$ [c]							IPV$_{B1}$ [c]			IPV$_{B2}$ [c]		
DPT		DPT$_1$	DPT$_2$	DPT$_3$							DPT$_{B1}$			DPT$_{B2}$		
HIB		HIB$_1$	HIB$_2$	HIB$_3$							HIB$_{B1}$					
PCV		PCV$_1$	PCV$_2$	PCV$_3$						PCV B$_1$						
RV		RV$_1$	RV$_2$	RV$_3$ [d]												
Influnza					IF$_1$ [e]	IF$_2$										
MMR							MMR$_1$			MMR$_2$				MMR$_3$		
TCV					TCV											
HAV								HAV$_1$				HAV$_2$ [f]				
Varicella										V1		V$_2$ [g]				
Tdap^h/Td															Tdap	
HPV															HPV1,2 [i]	HPV1,2,3 [j]
MCV^k							MCV1	MCV2								
JE								JE1	JE2							
Cholera								Ch1	Ch2							
PPSV23																
Rabies																
Yellow F																

Recommended Age   Catch-up Age Range   Vaccine for special Situations

a: Within 24 h after birth; **b:** Extra dose permitted in combination vaccine; **c:** can be given as combination vaccine,
d: not required for RV1; **e:** preferably pre-monsoon, then single dose annually till 5 years age: **f:** Single dose for live vaccine;
g: Second dose after 3-6 mo; **h:** after 7 yrs age if second DPT booster not received, else single dose at 10-12 yr, Use Td, if Tdap not available;
i: Two doses < 14 years, 6 mo apart.; **j:** Three doses after 14 years or in immunocompromized persons
k: Menactra® is approved as 2-doses between 9-23 mo at 3 months interval, Menveo® as single dose only after 2 yrs of age.

- IAP recommends a *booster dose of HIB at 16-18 months*, which is not included in NIS.

- IAP recommends *three doses of MMR at 9 months, 15 months and 4-6 years* instead of 2 doses of MR (no MMR) at 9-12 mo and 16-24 months in NIS.

- IAP also prescribes catch-up immunization of children above 5 years, while NIS is focused on children below 5 years.

Figure 5.1 provides a reference to the recommended ages for different vaccinations along with permitted age-group for catch-up doses, as per IAP recommendation.

5.3: MISSED (CATCH-UP) IMMUNIZATION

According to NFHS-IV data 2016, immunization coverage in India for all doses of UIP vaccines was merely ~62%, well below the targets of universal immunization. For individual vaccines, coverage varied from lowest of 63% for HBV and highest of 91% for BCG. Thus, a substantial number of children miss their vaccinations on due ages and need to be immunized at earliest possible opportunity. Following principles should be followed for catch-up immunization -

- Catch-up schedule for a child who had missed all or some of the vaccine doses must be tailored to achieve age-appropriate immunization as early as possible with minimum number of visits, but without compromising basic principles e.g. minimum dose interval etc.

- Upper age limit for catch-up immunization varies with the individual vaccines, determined by the need and safety issues and must be strictly followed.

- Multiple vaccines may be clubbed together in same visit to reduce the catch-up time. More than one inactivated vaccines, with or without a live vaccine can be given simultaneously or at any interval between them. However, two live vaccines should either be given simultaneously or at least 4 weeks apart.

- Partially immunized children should re-start catch-up immunization from the dose which was missed earlier *and not afresh*, irrespective of the period lapsed.

NIS permits catch-up immunization till the specified age-limits for individual vaccines (**Table 5.1**), using same number/s and interval of doses as for routine immunization. These age limits and dosage schedules have been decided for programmatic reasons - to cover most vulnerable population with available resources and use a simplified uniform schedule which can be delivered through public resources.

IAP recommendations for catch-up immunization are based largely on scientific basis and hence, might differ from NIS. Upper age limits are usually higher in IAP schedule except for RV vaccines and dosage schedules may differ from those used for routine immunization.

Table 5.3 presents IAP recommendations for Catch-up immunization with various vaccines. Some important details (with NIS recommendations in italics) are as follows –

BCG is recommended till 5 years of age (*vs 1 yr in NIS*) without prior Tuberculin testing, at earliest opportunity.

Polio vaccination is recommended till 5 years with –

- Three doses of IM-IPV at 0, 1, 6 months in fully unimmunized children, though two doses, instead of three, may be used at minimum 8 weeks interval.
- Children born after switch from tOPV to bOPV (25 April, 2016), who have not received IPV in the past, should also receive one dose of IM-IPV at earliest opportunity.
- *NIS recommends total 3 doses of OPV at monthly interval till five years of age for catch-up immunization. fIPV is given only till one year of age with first and last dose.*

DPT vaccination is recommended till the 18 years of age, with choice of vaccine depending on the age and previous immunization status –

- *Fully unimmunized children below 7 years* of age require three primary doses of DTwP at 0, 1 and 6 months, followed by a booster dose after 6 months of last primary dose. Second booster is not required, if the last dose was received beyond the age of 4 years.

- *Partly-immunized children below 7 years* must re-start from the dose which was missed *and not afresh*, irrespective of the period lapsed. 5-year Booster is not needed if the last dose was received after 4 years of age.

- *Fully unimmunized children above 7 years* of age are recommended a single dose of Tdap followed by two doses of Td at 0,1 and 6 months. DTwP vaccine should not be used beyond 7 years of age due to increased risk of side effects.

- *Partly-immunized children above 7 years* must receive a single dose of Tdap followed by Td after one month, if required. To complete total three doses of a tetanus containing vaccine, including the previous dose.

- *NIS provides primary DPT doses as pentavalent vaccine till 1 year only, though boosters may be given upto 7 years of age.*

HBV vaccination is recommended with no age limit as –

- Three-doses at 0, 1, 6 month for catch-up immunization. Combination vaccine with HAV may be used.

- Partially immunized children must re-start catch-up doses from the dose which was missed and *not afresh*, irrespective of period lapsed, to complete total 3 doses.

- Pre-vaccination antibody screening is not recommended except in contact of an HBsAg positive case.

- *NIS recommends HBV as pentavalent vaccine till 1 year only with same schedule i.e. three doses at 0, 1, 2 months.*

HIB vaccination is recommended till 5 years, with –

- Age-wise schedule i.e. Two doses at one month interval below one year (6-12 months), and single dose after one year. A booster dose after 8 weeks of last/single dose is recommended only in children <15 months of age.

- *NIS provides HIB as pentavalent vaccine till 1 year only with same dosage schedule of 0, 1, 2 months.*

PCV vaccination is recommended till 5 years with -

- Age-wise schedule i.e. Two doses at one month interval during 6-23 months of age with a booster in second year if the last dose was given before 1 year. Children above two years of age are advised only one dose of PCV13 or two doses of PCV10 at 8 weeks interval, without booster.

- *NIS provides PCV vaccination only till 1 year, with two doses at 8 weeks interval and a Booster at 9-12 months.*

Rotavirus vaccination should not be initiated -

- Beyond 15 weeks of age as per IAP recommendations due to insufficient safety data and all doses must be completed by 32 weeks. Vaccination should be avoided, if age of the infant is uncertain.

- *Beyond one year of age as per NIS. However if the first dose was received before 12 months of age, two subsequent doses may be given at monthly interval even after the first year, to complete the course.*

MMR vaccination after infancy involves –

- Two doses of MMR at least four weeks apart, with no upper age limit.
- Pregnancy should be excluded before vaccination in adolescent girls, due to potential risk of Congenital Rubella syndrome.
- Children, who received MMR-1 at 9-12 months but missed the second dose at 15-18 months, must receive two doses of MMR at minimum 4 weeks interval. Combination MMRV vaccine may be used in children 4-12 years of age with two doses at 6-12 weeks interval.

- *Under NIS, MR vaccine is provided till 5 years of age with two doses at four weeks interval.*

Japanese encephalitis vaccination is recommended–

- Till 18 years of age by IAP, with two doses of inactivated vaccines at one month interval.
- *Till 15 years of age in NIS, with two doses of Live attenuated vaccine at one month interval, in endemic districts.*

HAV vaccination has no upper age limit with –

- Two doses of inactivated vaccine 6-18 months apart *or* a single dose of Live Vaccine in children *or* combined HAV & HBV vaccine with three-dose at 0, 1, 6 months in previously HBV unimmunized children.
- Partly immunized children who have received only one dose of inactivated HAV, must receive second dose to complete two-dose schedule.
- IAP recommends pre-vaccination screening for HAV antibodies in children above 10 years, due to high chance of natural infection with > 50% seropositivity by this age.

Varicella vaccination is recommended till 18 years of age without evidence of immunity i.e. documented vaccination, history of disease or laboratory evidence, with two doses at 3 months interval if <13 years or 4-8 weeks interval if >13 years. However, all high-risk children should receive two doses 4–8 weeks apart irrespective of age.

Influenza vaccination is recommended to all children below 5 years (and in high-risk children beyond this age) with two doses of inactivated vaccine at 4-week interval in first year, followed by single dose annually before peak season.

Typhoid vaccination is recommended up to 18 years of age, preferably with a single dose of TCV (even in those who have received TPSV earlier – with 4 weeks interval). However, TPSV may also be considered above 2 years of age with a single dose every three years.

Table 5.3: Catch-up immunization for fully unimmunized persons (IAP)		
Vaccine	**Age limit (for only or last dose)**	**Schedule**
BCG	5 yr	Single dose
DPT	None	Age <7 yr: Three doses as DTwP/DTaP at 0, 1, 6 mo, B after 6 mo[1] Age >7 yr: Three doses as Tdap >Td >Td at 0, 1, 6 mo
IPV	5 yr	Three doses at 0, 1, 6 mo *or* Two doses at 0, 2 mo *or* Single dose, if born after 25.4.2016 and received bOPV only.
HBV	None	Three doses at 0,1,6 mo
HIB	5 yr	*Age 6–12 mo:* Two doses at 0, 1 mo, Booster after 8 weeks Age 12–15 mo: Single dose, Booster after 8 weeks Age 15 mo - 5 yr: Single dose, No booster
RV	32 wks	Two/Three doses at monthly interval[2]
PCV	5 years	Age <6 mo: Three doses at 0, 1, 2 mo, Booster 6 mo after last dose Age 6-12 mo: Two doses at 0, 1 mo, Booster in second year Age >12-23 mo: two doses at 0, 1 mo, No Booster Age >23 mo: Two dose PCV 10 (0, 2 mo) or Single dose PCV 13, No booster
MMR[3]	Nil	Two doses at 0, 1 mo
JE	18 years	Two doses at 0, 3 mo
HAV[4]	Nil	Two doses at 0, 6 mo (Inactivated HIV), *or* Single dose (Live HAV)
Varicella	18 yr	<13 yr: Two doses, 0, 3 mo >13 yr: two doses, 0-1 mo
Typhoid	18 yr	TPSV single dose every 3 years, *or* TCV single dose

[1] If last dose was given before 4 years
[2] RV *immunization* should not be initiated beyond 15 weeks of age and all doses must be completed by 32 weeks.
[3] Exclude Pregnancy before vaccination in adolescent girls, due to potential risk of CRS.
[4] Pre-vaccination screening recommended at 10 years

5.4: ADOLESCENT IMMUNIZATION

Many children remain unimmunized or partially immunized till they reach adolescence. Parental enthusiasm to get their children immunized often wanes with advancing age of the child and late-boosters are frequently missed. Recent years have witnessed rising incidence of vaccine-preventable diseases in adolescents due to missed boosters and shift of the age-epidemiology towards older age groups.

Adolescence offers an opportunity to fulfill these childhood immunization gaps as well as to improve herd immunity, reducing susceptible population and disease transmission. Adolescent immunization also aims to – a) protect against diseases with higher morbidity during adolescence e.g. Hepatitis A, Varicella; b) boost the waning immunity of early childhood vaccines e.g. DPT, c) counter upward shift of age-epidemiology following expanding childhood immunizations; and d) provide vaccines more relevant in adolescent age groups e.g. HPV or vaccines for travelers going abroad for studies. Catch-up vaccination of adolescent girls not only protects them but also offers some protection to their prospective offsprings from diseases like Pertussis and Congenital Rubella syndrome.

Vaccines recommended for the Adolescent immunization include (**Table 5.4**) –

a) Vaccines, missed in early childhood (Catch-up immunization);

b) Vaccines, against diseases common in or after adolescence e.g. HPV.

c) Vaccines, to be used in special circumstances.

Table 5.4: Adolescent Immunization	
A) Age-specific Adolescent immunization	
HPV (in Females)	Age-9-14 yrs: Two doses at 0 and 6 months Age >14 yrs: Three doses at 0, 1/2, 6 months
Tdap	Single dose followed by Td every 10 years[1]
B) Catch-up Childhood Immunization (to complete total...)	
MMR	Two doses at 4-8 weeks interval
HBV	Three doses at 0, 1 and 6 months
HAV	Two doses at 0 and 6 months
TCV	Single dose
Varicella	Two doses at 4-8 weeks interval
Japanse Encephalitis	Two doses at 0-3 months (in endemic districts)
C) Adolescent immunizations in special circumstances	
Influenza	Single dose every year, in high risk cases
PCV/PPSV	Single dose PCV13 followed by PPSV after 8 weeks[2]
Rabies vaccine	Post-exposure prophylaxis

[1] Adolescents, who are not immunized with DPT previously, must receive two further doses of Td at one and six month interval to complete catch-up vaccination, recommended till the 18 years of age.
[2] Repeat PPSV once only after 5 years, if high-risk state continues.

Frequently Asked Questions (FAQs)

1. **Why do IAP recommendations differ from National Immunization schedule?**

    NIS is the most practical but not necessarily an ideal schedule, with an aim to cover most vulnerable population with available resources and to use a simplified uniform schedule which can be delivered through public resources. Many useful vaccines have been left-out in NIS and dosages schedules have been tailored to minimize number of visits due to cost and logistic considerations. IAP recommendations are based on the current scientific knowledge and revised time to time. Accordingly, these recommendations are more appropriate and updated, but may be difficult to implement through public resources.

2. **What is meant by recommended age of vaccination?**

The recommended age in weeks/months/years means completed weeks/months/years.

3. **What is a *valid dose*? A child was given MR vaccine at the beginning of the 9th month (just after completing 8 months). Whether it should be acceptable?**

Vaccine doses administered up to 4 days before the due date can be counted as valid (exception rabies). If a dose is administered ≥ 5 days before, it is considered as invalid dose and needs to be repeated. Accordingly, MR vaccine needs to be repeated in this case after due date, preferably after four weeks of invalid dose.

4. **A child was given second dose of Pentavalent vaccine after 15 days of first dose, by mistake. What should be done?**

If given less than four weeks apart, second dose should be repeated, at least 4 weeks after the invalid dose.

5. **What is generally meant by vaccination at birth?**

Vaccination at birth means as early as possible within 24 to 72 hours after birth or at least not later than one week after birth.

6. **What is meant by "same day vaccination"?**

Simultaneous or Same-day vaccination implies administration of 2 or more vaccines at the same time or within the same immunization session (about 6 hours).

7. **Whether more than one vaccine can be given on same day ? If not, then what should be the ideal time interval between different vaccines?**

Any number of vaccines can be given on the same day as immune system is capable to interact with millions of antigen together, without interference. In fact, combination vaccines are as effective as separate vaccinations.

However, two live vaccines should be given either simultaneously or at least 4 weeks apart, as ongoing immune process for previous vaccine might interfere with uptake of subsequent vaccine. This rule does not apply to more than one inactivated vaccines (with/without a live vaccine), which can be given simultaneously or at any interval between doses.

8. **Whether a home-delivered child can be given BCG, OPV and HBV at 1 month of age?**

Upper age limits for birth doses of OPV and HBV are 15 days and 24 hours respectively and the purpose of giving these doses is lost, if delayed beyond this period. BCG may be given at any age, though it is preferable to club it with primary doses at 6-week, to minimize number of visits. Subsequent immunizations should continue, as scheduled.

9. **If a child is brought late for a subsequent dose, should one re-start with the first dose of a vaccine?**

No, it should be started from the dose which was missed.

For example, If a child who has received BCG, Penta-1, OPV-1 and RV-1 at 6 weeks, returns at 11 months of age, s/he must begin with Penta-2, OPV-2, RV-2 and MR-1, along with JE-1 (if applicable).

10. **If a totally unimmunized child presents at 11 months of age, whether all due vaccines can be given together on the same day?**

Yes, all due vaccines (BCG, Penta-1, OPV-1, fIPV-1, RV-1*, MR-1 and JE (if applicable) can be given in the same sitting. However, injections should preferably be given on different sides or at least one inch apart, if it is necessary to give two injections on same limb. (*Note that IAP does not recommend first dose of RV beyond 15 weeks and any dose beyond 32 weeks, though recommended upto one year in NIS)*

11. A fully or partly unimmunized child presents at three years of age. Which vaccines are to be given?

RV vaccine is not given above 1 year. All other vaccines, recommended for routine immunization under IAP schedule are indicated in this child, though the immunization schedule must be tailored accordingly to previous immunization history and catch-up immunization schedule discussed earlier (**Table 5.3**), with an aim to complete all immunizations as early as possible with minimum number of visits.

12. Which vaccines must be given to a child above 5 years of age who has never been vaccinated?

BCG, IPV/OPV, HIB, PCV and RV are not recommended beyond 5 years for healthy children. For age-appropriate schedules of other vaccines in cases of missed immunization, see **Table 5.3**.

References

1. Ministry of Health and Family welfare, Government of India. National Immunization Schedule *In:* Immunization Handbook for health workers 2018; pp 67-78.
2. Kasi SG et al. IAP Advisory Committee on Vaccines and Immunization Practices (ACVIP): Recommended Immunization Schedule (2020-21) and Update on Immunization for Children Aged 0 Through 18 Years. Indian Pediatrics 2021; 58: 44-53.
3. Chatterjee P. Scheduling of vaccines. *In:* IAP Guidebook on Immunization 2018-19 - Advisory Committee on Vaccines and Immunization Practices, Indian Academy of Pediatrics, 3rd Edition, New Delhi, Jaypee Brothers 2020; pp 84-91.
4. Aggarwal A et al. Vaccination Schedules. *In:* Vashishtha V et al. FAQs on Vaccines and immunization practices. 2nd Edition. New Delhi, Jaypee Brothers 2015; pp 32-40.
5. Chatterjee P. Immunization of Adolescents. *In:* IAP Guidebook on Immunization 2018-19 - Advisory Committee on Vaccines and Immunization Practices, Indian Academy of Pediatrics, 3rd Edition, New Delhi, Jaypee Brothers 2020; pp 396-403.
6. Bansal CP et al. Adolescent Immunization *In:* Vashishtha V et al. FAQs on Vaccines and immunization practices. 2nd Edition. New Delhi, Jaypee Brothers 2015; pp 85-98.

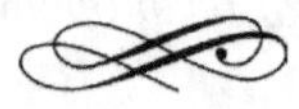

Adverse Events following Immunization

All vaccines are extremely, but not absolutely, safe and adverse reactions are rare but do occur after immunizations either due to the vaccine *per se* or due to the process of vaccination.

Adverse event following immunization (AEFI) is defined as *"an untoward medical occurrence which follows immunization though does not necessarily have a causal relationship with the usage of the vaccine."* It may present as any - a) unfavorable or unintended sign, b) abnormal laboratory finding, c) symptom, or d) disease.

6.1: CLASSIFICATIONS

AEFI are classified according to the probable cause, frequency and severity. For the programmatic purpose, AEFIs are classified according to probable cause, as follows:

Cause-wise AEFI are classified (2015) as follows -

1. *Vaccine-product related reaction,* due to inherent property of the vaccine product, e.g. VAPP following OPV or febrile seizure following DPT vaccination (**Table 6.1**).

2. *Vaccine-quality defect related reaction,* due to qualitative defect/s in the vaccine or its delivery device provided by manufacturer, e.g. insufficient inactivation of the virus (IPV), leading to disease (Poliomyelitis). These reactions are very rare due to adoption of good manufacturing practices (WHO-GMP) by manufacturers.

3. *Immunization-error related reaction* (programmatic errors), due to - a) inappropriate handling e.g. cold-chain issues, b) inappropriate prescribing e.g. ignoring contraindica-

Vaccine	Local Reactions	Minor Systemic reactions	Serious AEFI (with usual time limit)	Risk for serious AE
BCG	90-95%	-	BCG adenitis (2-6 mo)	1-10/10000
	-	-	BCG Osteitis (1-12 mo)	1-700/ million
	-	-	Disseminated TB (1-12 mo)	0.2-1.5/ million
OPV	-	<1%	VAPP (4-30 days)*	2-4/ million
HBV	5%	<6%	Anaphylaxis (0-1hr)	10/ million
HIB	5-15%	2-10%	-	-
Penta	Upto 50%	Upto 55%	Inconsolable cry (0-24 hrs)	<1/100
	-	-	Seizures (0-3 days)	<1/100
	-	-	HHE (0-24 hrs)	<1-2/1000
	-	-	Anaphylaxis (0-1 hr)	1-2/million
	-	-	Encephalopathy (0-2 days)	<1/million
RV	-	-	Intussception (3-14 days)	1-2/lac
PCV	20%	20%	HHE (0-24 hrs)	<0.01%
			Seizures (0-3 days)	<0.01%
MR/MMR	10%	5-15%	Febrile Seizures (6-12 days)	3/1000
	-	-	Thrombocytopenia (15-35 days)	1/30000
JE	1-3%	5-10%	-	-
TT/Td	10%	10-25%	Branchial neuritis (2-28 days)	5-10/million
	-	-	Anaphylaxis (0-1 hr)	1-2/million

* 4-75 days in contacts

tions, c) inappropriate administration e.g. use of wrong vaccine/diluents or unsafe injection practices. Injection abscess, regional nerve injury and toxic shock syndrome following measles vaccination are common examples of immunization errors.

4. *Immunization-anxiety related reactions*, are more common during mass vaccination campaigns and in older children due to fear or pain of injection rather than due to the vaccine. These reactions often present as fainting, dizziness, perioral tingling etc. Younger children may present with breath-holding spells, sometimes leading to transient unconsciousness or seizure-like activity.

5. *Coincidental events*, due to something other than the above factors with a chance association, e.g. fever after vaccination in a child with pre-existing upper respiratory infection. Considering the sheer number of children immunized, specially during mass immunizations, these events are inevitable, often erroneously attributed to immunization.

Frequency-wise AEFI are classified as - *Very common*(>10%), *common* (1–10%), *uncommon* (0.1–1.0%), *rare* (0.01–0.1%) and *very rare* (<0.01%). **Table 6.1** provides incidence of common product-related adverse events following vaccines included in NIS.

Severity-wise AEFI are classified as:

1. *Serious AEFI if results in – a)* death, b) hospitalization, c) significant disability including birth defects, or d) require intervention to prevent permanent damage, e.g. anaphylaxis, seizures, intussusception, etc. AEFI which occur in clusters or cause major parental/community concern are also be considered as serious.

2. *Severe AEFI* are those which are of relatively minor medical significance but perceived to be severe in terms of intensity, e.g. high fever following DPT or swelling

extending beyond nearest joint. Patient does not require hospitalization or is not left with a sequelae.

3. *Minor vaccine reactions* are common, presenting as *local reactions*, e.g. pain swelling, redness etc. at the injection site or *systemic reactions*, e.g. fever, irritability, malaise or others, e.g. rash after measles vaccine or keloid scar after BCG. These reactions can be managed without any specific treatment or reassurance and usually resolve within 2-3 days. Some of these reaction may be due to adjuvants, stabilizers and preservatives in the vaccine rather than the antigen.

Clinically, AEFRs may present immediately or after many days, with:

1. *Local reactions*: e.g. pain, erythema and induration. These reactions are more common with whole cell pertussis vaccines and aluminum adjuvanted vaccines. *Frequency of local reactions tends to increase with subsequent doses.* These reactions may be partly ameliorated by ice application and paracetamol.

2. *Systemic reactions:* Fever is the most common systemic reaction, more common with whole cell pertussis vaccines and aluminum-adjuvanted vaccines. *Systemic reactions tend to decline with increasing age and increasing number of doses.* Although prophylactic paracetamol may reduce the incidence of post-vaccine febrile reactions, it has been found to blunt immune responses of some vaccines and should be used judiciously. Post- vaccine fever rarely last for >48 hours and any fever persisting beyond this time should be evaluated for other causes.

3. *Allergic reactions* are rare and may present with variable severity, ranging from mild urticaria to life-threatening anaphylaxis. These reactions are rarely due to the vaccine antigen, usually caused by other vaccine constituents, e.g. residual animal protein (egg), stabilizers or preservatives (thiomersol) etc. Since occurrence of anaphylaxis cannot be predicted in most cases, all vaccinees should be

observed for 15-30 minutes. Children with history of serious allergy to any of the vaccine constituents should not receive the vaccine.

6.2: ANAPHYLAXIS

Anaphylaxis is very rare (<1-2/million doses) but most feared and life-threatening AEFI folliwing vaccinations. Many of these reactions are not due to antigens *per se* but due to excipients in formulations e.g. Neomycin, gelatin and egg proteins.

Clinically, anaphylaxis usually develops within 5–30 minutes of vaccination, though might develop even after 2-4 hours, presenting with sudden onset and rapid progression of multi-systemic manifestations involving at least two of three – Dermatological, Cardiovascular and respiratory systems.

Many cases die rapidly due to airway obstruction or cardio-respiratory arrest, unless treated immediately. Even after initial recovery, some patients may develop recurrence *(biphasic reaction)* after 1–8 hours and must be observed atleast for 24 hours.

Diagnosis of anaphylaxis depends on history of exposure and catastrophic clinical picture. Table 6.2 provides Brighton's diagnostic criteria for anaphylaxis following vaccinations with different levels of certainity (**Table 6.2**). Nearest differential diagnosis of Anaphylaxis in context of immunizations is vasovagal syncope or fainting spells, - an anxiety reaction, common in adolescent girls (**Table 6.3**).

Management: Anaphylaxis is a life-threatening emergency and all vaccination health workers must be trained to recognize and manage anaphylaxis in emergency.

Table 6.2: Diagnostic criteria for Anaphylaxis (Brighton criteria)

System	Major Criteria	Minor criteria
Dermatologic	• Gen Urticaria or Erythema • Gen or local Angioedema • Gen Pruritus with Rash	• Generalized pruritus without rash • Generalized prickle sensation • Localized injection site urticaria • Red and itchy eyes

Cardiovascular	• Measured hypotension *or*
	• Clinical shock (any three)
	  - Tachycardia
	  - Capillary refill time >3 Sec
	  - Reduced central pulse volume
	  - Decreased/ Loss of Consciousness
		• Clinical (any two)
		  - Tachycardia
		  - Capillary refill time >3 sec
		  - Hypotension
		  - Decreased consciousness

Respiratory	• Bilateral wheeze
	• Stridor
	• upper airway swelling
	• Resp distress (any two)
	  - Tachypnea
	  - Accessory muscle use
	  - Intercostal recession
	  - Cyanosis
	  - Grunting
		• Persistent dry cough
		• Hoarse voice
		• Difficult breathing without wheeze or stridor
		• Sensation of throat closure
		• Sneezing or Rhinorrhea

Gastrointestinal	-	• Diarrhoea • Abdominal pain • Nausea • Vomiting
Laboratory	-	Mast cell tryptase elevation > upper normal limit

Levels of Diagnostic certainty as per Brighton criteria -

Level 1: ≥ 1 Major dermatological criterion *with* ≥ 1 major CVS and/or Resp Criterion.

Level 2: ≥ 1 major CVS and/or Resp Criterion *with* >1 minor criteria from other systems (except CVS/Resp) **OR** ≥ 1major dermatological criteria *with* ≥ 1 minor CVS/RS criterion

Level 3: ≥ 1 minor CVS/RS criterion *with* ≥1 minor criterion from each of ≥ 2 different systems

Table 6.3: D/D Syncope *versus* Anaphylaxis		
	Fainting/syncope	**Anaphylaxis**
Onset after injection	Immediate	Usually after 5-30 min
Skin	Pale, sweaty, cold	Rash, swollen face/eyes
Breathing	Normal to deep	Noisy (airway obstruction)
Heart rate	Bradycardia	Tachycardia
Carotid Pulsations	Strong	Weak
Blood pressure	Normal/Transient ↓	Hypotension
Abdominal	Nausea/Vomiting	Abdominal cramps
Sensorium	Transient loss, Good response to prone position	Prolonged loss, No response to prone position

Immediate subcutaneous administration of *Adrenaline* 1:1000 solution (0.1 ml/kg; max 0.5 ml), is life-saving and should be administered at slightest suspicion without waiting for expert confirmation. All government vaccination sites are provided with *Anaphylaxis kit* containing Adrenaline, Insulin/tuberculin syringe, 24-25 G needle and instructions about age-wise doses – *0.05 ml < 1 year, 0.1 ml from 1-6 years and 0.2 ml from 6-12 years, 0.3 ml from 12-18 years and 0.5 ml in adults.*

SC Adrenaline may be repeated after 15 minutes, apart from other respiratory and cardiovascular supporting measures. All cases should be hospitalized for at least 24 hours to watch for late-phase reactions. Antihistamines and steroids have no role in the immediate management of anaphylaxis.

Prevention: Anaphylaxis is rare and unpredictable event, though all parents/children should be asked about the history of allergic reaction due to previous dose or any of the vaccine components e.g. neomycin, eggs etc before administration. All vaccinees should also be observed for 15-30 minutes after vaccination.

6.3: AEFI SURVEILLANCE: REPORTING, INVESTIGATION AND CAUSALITY ASSESSMENT

AEFI Surveillance is usually a passive system to enable spontaneous reporting of all adverse events to monitor safety of a licensed and marketed vaccine product, with special emphasis on known serious or new adverse events.

Reporting: Any health care provider, whether in public or private sector, who comes across any AEFI, must report it to local health authorities, specially in case of - a) Serious AEFI, e.g. death, hospitalization, cluster, disability; b) Signal and events associated with a newly introduced vaccine; c) AEFI, probably due to immunization-error related reactions; d) Significant events of unexplained cause within 30 days of immunization; and e) Event causing significant parental or community concern.

In the Government sector, health workers are asked to notify all serious and severe AEFIs immediately to the nearest primary health center medical officer (MO) or the District Immunization Officer (DIO). Private practitioners are also encouraged to notify AEFIs to Medical officer incharge of nearest Government health center.

Medical officer then reports basic details of the case in a structured Case reporting form (CRF) in 24 hours to the DIO, who has to verify the case within another 24 hours and send to the State Immunization officer as well as to Immunization Division, Ministry of Health and Family Welfare (MOHFW) simultaneously.

Investigation: As soon as an AEFI is reported, case investigation begins using preliminary case investigation format (PCIF) as a checklist. Investigation includes verifying personal details, vaccine and program details, clinical review and interviews of the health-care givers. to understand the sequence of events. An epidemiological investigation is also conducted along with assessment of cold chain and vaccine transportation conditions. In case of death, postmortem is recommended or verbal autopsies are done to find out the cause. PCIF with related investigation reports are submitted simultaneously to the state and the national level within 10 days of notification for causality assessment.

Causality assessment: Causality assessment is the systematic evaluation of the information collected on investigation to determine the likelihood of the event having been caused by the vaccines received. It is done at state and national level AEFI committee of experts within a month of receipt of all reports of the AEFI case.

Four major components of causality assessment process are - a) to ascertain eligibility of the case for Causality assessment, b) to evaluate available facts of the case on the basis of a check-list, c) to assess the strength of association on the basis of an algorithm, and d) To classify the case in pre-determined categories.

A case is eligible for causality assessment only if it has a valid diagnosis, which may be based on any standard literature definitions and may be a disease, symptom, sign or laboratory finding. Brighton's criteria, (available at *https://brightoncollaboration.org/*) a collaborative effort to provide standardized case definitions for common AEFIs, are frequently used to arrive at a valid diagnosis for this purpose.

Process of the causality assessment involves assessment of temporal relationship, biological plausibility, strength and consistency of association, consideration of alternate explanations and known relationships between AEFI and vaccine, using a check-list (**Table 6.4**) and flow-chart (**Fig. 6.1**). Causality assessment can also be done using a WHO software (*http://gvsi-aefi-tools.org/*).

Table 6.4: Checklist for causality assessment

Step 2: Event checklist

Check ✓ all boxes that apply   Y: Yes N: No UK: Unknown NA: Not applicable

I. Is there strong evidence for other causes?	Y	N	UK	NA	Remark
Does a clinical examination, or laboratory tests on the patient, confirm another cause?	☐	☐	☐	☐	
II. Is there a known causal association with the vaccine or vaccination?					
Vaccine product(s)					
Is there evidence in the literature that this vaccine(s) may cause the reported event even if administered correctly?	☐	☐	☐	☐	
Did a specific test demonstrate the causal role of the vaccine or any of the ingredients?	☐	☐	☐	☐	
Immunization error					
Was there an error in prescribing or non-adherence to recommendations for use of the vaccine (e.g. use beyond the expiry date, wrong recipient etc.)?	☐	☐	☐	☐	
Was the vaccine's physical condition (e.g. colour, turbidity, presence of foreign substances etc.) abnormal at the time of administration?	☐	☐	☐	☐	
Was there an error in vaccine constitution/preparation by the vaccinator (e.g. wrong product, wrong diluent, improper mixing, improper syringe filling etc.)?	☐	☐	☐	☐	
Was there an error in vaccine handling (e.g. a break in the cold chain during transport, storage and/or immunization session etc.)?	☐	☐	☐	☐	
Was the vaccine administered incorrectly (e.g. wrong dose, site or route of administration; wrong needle size etc.)?	☐	☐	☐	☐	
Immunization anxiety					
Could the event have been caused by anxiety about the immunization (e.g. vasovagal, hyperventilation or stress-related disorder)?	☐	☐	☐	☐	
II (time). If "yes" to any question in II, was the event within the time window of increased risk?					
Did the event occur within an appropriate time window after vaccine administration?	☐	☐	☐	☐	
III. Is there strong evidence against a causal association?					
Is there strong evidence against a causal association?	☐	☐	☐	☐	
IV. Other qualifying factors for classification					
Could the event occur independently of vaccination (background rate)?	☐	☐	☐	☐	
Could the event be a manifestation of another health condition?	☐	☐	☐	☐	
Did a comparable event occur after a previous dose of a similar vaccine?	☐	☐	☐	☐	
Was there exposure to a potential risk factor or toxin prior to the event?	☐	☐	☐	☐	
Was there acute illness prior to the event?	☐	☐	☐	☐	
Did the event occur in the past independently of vaccination?	☐	☐	☐	☐	
Was the patient taking any medication prior to vaccination?	☐	☐	☐	☐	
Is there a biological plausibility that the vaccine could cause the event?	☐	☐	☐	☐	

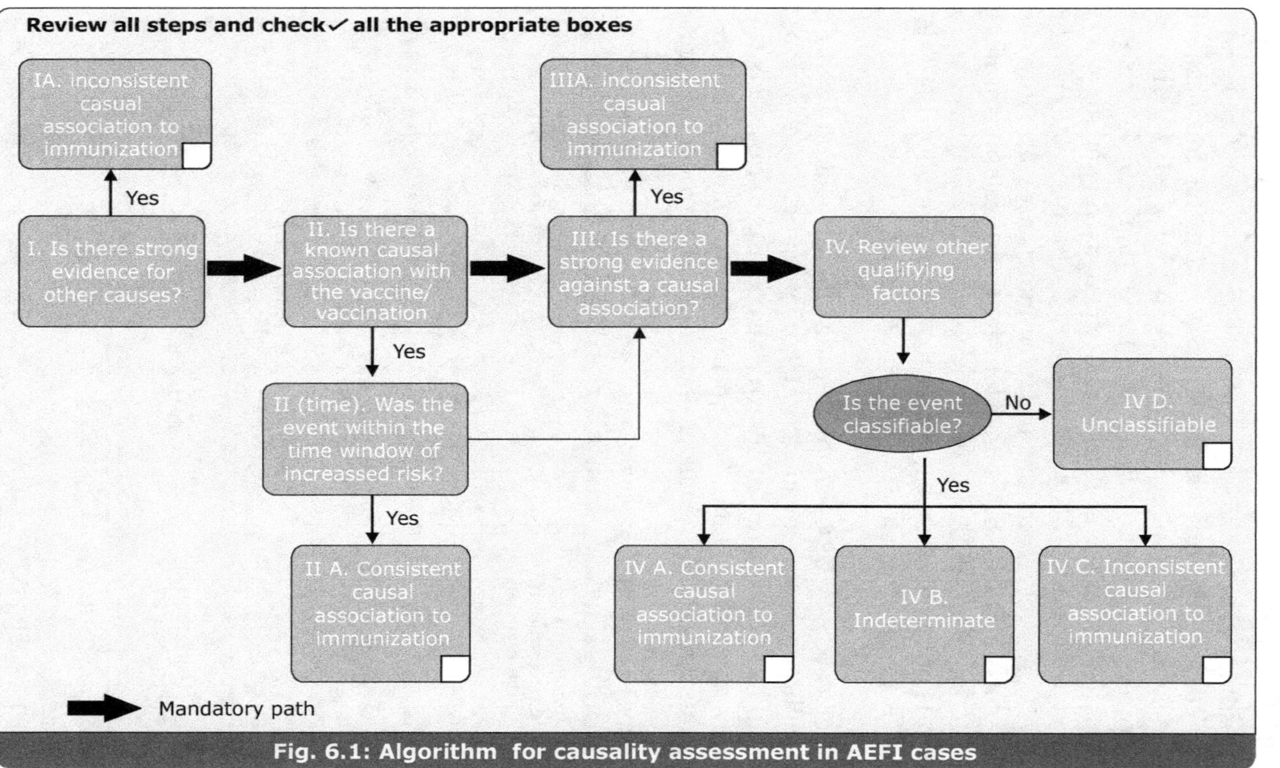

Fig. 6.1: Algorithm for causality assessment in AEFI cases

All reported AEFIs are investigated by specialists and classified (**Table 6.5**) causality-wise as – A) Consistent association, B) Indeterminate association, C) Inconsistent association i.e. coincidental events and D) Unclassifiable, if sufficient information is not available. (**Fig. 6.3**) Consistent causal association is further classified as related to - A1) Vaccine-Product, A2) Quality defect, A3) Immunization Error or A4) Anxiety reaction. Indeterminate cases arer further sub-classified as – B1) Consistent temporal relationship but with insufficient definitive evidence, and B2) Conflicting trends of consistency e.g. Thrombocytopenia following MR/MMR vaccination in a Dengue endemic area.

After causality assessment, the results are shared with all stakeholders for relevant action. For *product-related* reactions, regulator is informed if the frequency of AEFI exceeds the known baseline rate. For *quality-defect* related reactions, further analysis is needed to find out if a particular vaccine

Table 6.5: Causality Classification of AEFI

A. Consistent causal association to immunization	B. Indeterminate	C. Inconsistent causal association to immunization
• A1. Vaccine product-related reaction (as per published literature)	• B1. *Temporal relationship is consistent but there is insufficient definitie evidence for vaccine causing event (may be new vacine-linked event)	• C. Coincidental Underlying or emerging condition(s), or condition(s) caused by exposure to something other than vaccine
• A2. Vaccine quality defect-related reaction	• B2. Qualifying factors result in conflicting trends of consistency and inconsistency with causal association to immunization	
• A3. Immunization error-related reaction		
• A4. Immunization anxiety-related reaction		

• Unclassifiable	
Specify the additional information required for classification	

brand or lot is involved and the regulator and manufacturer needs to be informed. Immunization *error-related* reactions need reinforcement training of the staff and strengthening of supervision. When immunization *anxiety-related* reactions are identified, it should be ensured that the immunizations take place in a nonstressful environment.

All cases in the indeterminate category (B1) are maintained in a database and reviewed to identify a signal for causal association of the vaccine with a new AEFI. Cases in B2 are followed up for additional information which can help in making a decision to classify into vaccine/vaccination related or coincidental. Confirmation of classification of coincidental cases is conveyed to the informer and the patient and relatives. For unclassifiable cases, attempt is made to get the missing information for further classification, if possible.

Frequently Asked Questions (FAQs)

1. **Whether prophylactic paracetamol is advisable to all children receiving injectable vaccines e.g. DPT?**

    Antipyretics are commonly used to prevent or treat fever after vaccinations. However, some studies have shown blunting of the immune response in recipients of Post-vaccination Paracetamol. While further studies did not confirm such effect, WHO position paper 2015 recommends against use of prophylactic paracetamol due to lack of evidence of pain-mitigation effectiveness and/or the potential for altering vaccine effectiveness. However, Oral analgesics may be used therapeutically to mitigate pain and/ or fever linked to delayed reactogenicity.

2. **Which local reactions are considered as severe enough to require specific medical attention and reporting?**

    Transient local reactions are very common after injectable vaccines. specially those containing adjuvants. No specific treatment is required in most cases except local cold compresses, analgesics.e.g. paracetamol. However, Reactions with - a) Swelling extending beyond the nearest joint and/or b) Local pain/swelling/redness persisting for >3 days are considered as severe, requiring medical attention and must be reported.

3. **How does one identify and treat local cellulitis or abscess at the site of vaccination?**

Post-vaccination *Cellulitis* is defined as presence of local pain, erythema, induration and warmth (any three), which does not resolve rapidly and spontaneously or develops fluctuation. Post-vaccination *Abscess* denotes localized fluid collection at the site with fluctuation, which may rupture spontaneously or need surgical drainage. Fever and lymphadenopathy may or may not be present in both cases.

Cellultis needs to be treated with anti-inflammatory agents and local compresses, with or without antibiotics. Surgical drainage is essential for abscesses. Abscesses may be sterile or culture-positive. Antibiotics are not required for sterile abscesses.

4. **What are the early symptoms of Brachial neuritis after vaccination in upper arm?**

Brachial neuritis may present with a deep, steady and often severe aching pain over shoulder and upper arm followed in days or weeks with weakness and wasting of the shoulder or arm muscles. Sensory involvement may or may not be present.

5. **How can we differentiate an anaphylaxis reaction following vaccination from the fainting spell or syncope, a common immunization-anxiety reaction?**

While it is sometimes difficult to differentiate these two adverse events, features depicted in *table 6.3*, may be helpful.

6. **What are the presentation of Toxic-shock syndrome?**

Toxic-shock syndrome (TSS) is an acute life-threatening complication following use of contaminated vaccines which do not contain preservatives e.g. MR/MMR, and used after 3-6 hours of reconstitution with unsafe storage conditions. TSS is caused by an exotoxin TSS-1, usually released by staphylococci phage type-I.

Clinically, TSS is characterized by three *major* features: (i) sudden onset of high fever, (ii) severe hypotension/ shock and (iii) generalized erythematous rash after 24 hours of fever. Important *minor* features include—(a) mucosal lesions, e.g. strawberry tongue, conjunctival congestion, (b) vomiting/diarrhea, (c) severe myalgia, (d) altered sensorium without focal signs, (e) liver/renal abnormalities and (f) thrombocytopenia.

Diagnosis depends on presence of *all major criteria and/or minimum three minor criteria* after exclusion of other causes and negative blood culture.

Treatment includes drainage of infected site if required, parenteral antibiotics including vancomycin and supportive treatment for shock and other complications. Prognosis is poor in untreated cases. Appropriately treated cases recover in 7–10 days, leaving behind a desquamating lesion, especially over palm and soles.

7. **Whether All AEFIs, including minor side effects, needs to be reported and investigated?**

Although there is no restriction to report any suspected adverse event, including minor one, following are considered as more significant and investigated – a) Serious AEFI, e.g. death, hospitalization, cluster, disability; b) Signal and events associated with a newly introduced vaccine; c) AEFI, probably due to immunization-error related reactions; d) Significant events of unexplained cause within 30 days of immunization; and e) Event causing significant parental or community concern.

8. **Who can report an AEFI?**

Any health care provider, whether in public or private sector, who comes across any serious or severe AEFIs or others mentioned in FAQ1, must report it to nearest primary health center medical officer or the District Immunization officer. Private practitioners are also encouraged to notify them to local authorities. Medical officers then report basic details of the case in a more structured Case Report Form (CRF).

9. Whether there is any time-limit to report an AEFI after vaccination?

Although an AEFI may be reported anytime, usually an event within 30 days of vaccination is considered as more significant and investigated (Exceptions e.g. VAPP).

10. Whether there is any time-limit to consider an AEFI related to a vaccine?

Although some AEFIs may develop any time after vaccination, experience and guidelines suggest appropriate time windows for many AEFIs and occurrence of an event outside this window is considered as less significant. **Table 6.1** has given appropriate time windows for common AEFI e.g. less than 1 hour for anaphylaxis or 15-35 days for MMR-induced thrombocytopenia. However, the AEFIs can develop outside these time limits and need to be assessed in individual cases.

References

1. Ministry of Health and Family welfare, Government of India. Adverse Events Following Immunization: Surveillance and Response Operational Guidelines. New Delhi: 2015.
2. World Health Organization. Causality assessment of adverse event following immunization (AEFI): User manual for the revised WHO classification. 2013.
3. Prajapati BS. Adverse events following immunization, vaccine safety and misinformation against vaccination. *In:* Vashishtha V et al. FAQs on Vaccines and immunization practices. 2nd Edition. New Delhi, Jaypee brothers 2015; pp 63-75.
4. Pemde H. Adverse events following immunization. *In:* IAP Guidebook on Immunization 2018-19 - Advisory Committee on Vaccines and Immunization Practices, Indian Academy of Pediatrics, 3rd Edition, New Delhi, Jaypee Brothers 2020; pp 69-83.
5. Ministry of Health and Family welfare, Government of India. Adverse events following Immunization. *In:* Immunization Handbook for health workers 2018; pp 107-126.

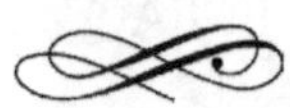

Section

II

Vaccines included in National Immunization Schedule

BCG Vaccine

Recent years have witnessed global resurgence of tuberculosis due to spread of HIV infection and emergence of multi-drug resistance. Vaccination is the integral part of WHO's *"End TB strategy"*, targetted to bring down the incidence of newly diagnosed cases by 80% and mortality by 90%, by the year 2030.

Vaccine: BCG (*Bacille Calmette-Guérin*) *vaccine* is the oldest among currently used vaccines*, developed in 1921 at the Pasteur Institute by French microbiologist *Leon Charles Albert Calmette* and veterinary surgeon *Camille Guérin*. In India, it has been used for mass vaccination since 1948. (*Earliest vaccine was smallpox, developed in 1798).

Contents & Storage: BCG is a live attenuated vaccine derived from many strains of the Mycobacterium bovis, commonest being the *Danish 1331 strain*, which is also used in India. Other commonly used strains include *Tokyo 172-1* and *Russian BCG-I* strains. Each vaccine is prepared from lyophilized seed lots of strain preserved by WHO and end-product should fulfill WHO standards. Each dose contains between $1x10^6$ and $33x10^6$ Colony Forming Units (CFU) with Glutamate as stabilizer.

BCG (Tubervac®) is supplied as a freeze-dried powder in multi-dose vials along with a diluent (Sodium chloride) and needs to be reconstituted before use.

Being heat & light sensitive, BCG comes in dark glass vials and must be stored in a dark place. While unopened vials can be stored at 2-8°C for up to 24 months, reconstituted vaccine must be used within 4-6 hours, till then kept in 2-8°C, away from light. On improper storage or longer use of opened vial, vaccine not only loses its potency (live vaccine) but is also at risk of bacterial contamination (does not contain preservative).

Dosage & administration: In NIS, BCG is given intradermally over the left shoulder as 0.05 ml at birth or in newborns and as 0.1 ml in infants above one month. However, WHO and most manufacturers recommend 0.05 ml dose till 1 year of age.

Considering the small volume, BCG must be given with a tuberculin syringe and 26 gauge needle. Site should be cleaned only with sterile cotton swab and not with spirit or alcohol (FAQ 2), which may affect the viability of bacilli. Technique of Intradermal injection is important, which should raise a wheal of ~5 mm over injection site, lasting for 15-20 minutes.

Immunization Schedule: BCG must be given at birth for all institutional deliveries including healthy preterms or at earliest contact. Vaccination at birth means as early as possible within 24 to 72 hours or at least not later than one week after birth. However, it can also be given at 6 weeks of age with other due vaccines if missed at birth e.g. in home deliveries..

Catch-up immunization is permitted till one year of age under NIS, though IAP and WHO recommends it till 5 years without preceding tuberculin testing.

Efficacy: BCG protects largely by inducing *cell mediated immunity* rather than the humoral immunity. Protective value is highly controversial, though generally accepted as ~70-90% against severe disease e.g. military or neurotuberculosis and ~50-60% against pulmonary tuberculosis. Protection declines over time, dropping <10% after 10-15 years.

It is generally assumed that BCG, though protecting against tubercular disease, does not prevent primary infection. However a recent meta-analysis (Roy et al, 2014)[6] found that BCG-vaccinated children exposed to open contacts had 19% lesser infection than unvaccinated children, suggesting modest protective effect against infection as well.

Safety: Following BCG administration, local wheel subsides after 15-20 min and nothing is visible at the site for 2-3 weeks before development of an progressively enlarging indurated papule of 4-8 mm. Subsequently, this papule ulcerates by ~6-8 weeks (sometimes covered with a crust), before forming a tiny round scar of 2-10 mm size by 6-12 weeks. Some papules do not ulcerate at all, while other may ulcerate many times, before eventual scarring. These changes at the site of vaccination are natural course of vaccination and should not be construed as side effects.

True side-effects are rare and include -

1. *Local reactions,* including secondary infection or keloid formation at the site of injection may develop in 1:1000 – 1:10000 vaccinees despite correct administration. Frequency of local reactions depend on many factors including the strain used in the vaccine, number of viable bacilli in the batch, and variation in injection technique. *Danish strain, used in Indian vaccines is more reactogenic than others.*

2. *Regional Lymphadenitis:* Transient enlargement of the ipsilateral regional lymph nodes (usually axillary) is not uncommon, though these nodes remain small (<1 cm),

do not adhere to overlying skin and regress eventually without any intervention.

BCG lymphadenitis (BCGitis) after 4–8 weeks of vaccination (as late as 11 months), due to lymphatic spread of viable bacilli to the regional nodes, has been reported in 3-10/1000 vaccinees. It may be *non-suppurative* with enlargement of regional lymphnode/s without signs of inflammation or *suppurative* with development of fluctuation and erythema. Lesions are on same side of vaccination without constitutional symptoms and normal chest skiagram. FNAC may reveal AFB due to presence of bovine vaccine bacilli and should not be misconstrued as tubercular disease.

3. **Disseminated disease (BCGiosis)** is extremely rare (1-4/ million doses) except in immunocompromized children and presents usually after 6-12 months with lesions distal to the site of inoculation e.g. skin (Scrofuloderma, Tuberculids), bones (osteitis or osteomyelitis) or intestines. Children with HIV or other cellular immunodeficiency disorders e.g. severe combined immunodeficiency etc. are more likely to develop disseminated disease, as common as in 1%.

4. **Immune reconstitution inflammatory syndrome (IRIS)** may present as local abscess at the site of BCG vaccination/scar or regional lymphadenitis within 6-12 weeks of starting antiretrovital therapy in HIV and immune reconstitution. Disseminated disease is extremely unlikely. Other very rare but notable BCG syndromes with immunological basis include uveitis, optic neuritis, sarcoidosis and skin lesions e.g. lupus vulgaris and erythema nodosum,

Contraindications: There are no absolute contraindications, except:

1. Congenital immunodeficiency disorders.

2. Acquired immunodeficiency, e.g. AIDS* or malignancy (*see FAQ 16).

3. Immunosuppressive therapy i.e. steroids, chemotherapy or radiotherapy, including infants exposed to immunosuppressive therapy *in utero* or via breastfeeding.

In cases with local eczema or dermatological disease, it may be given on other side.

Frequently Asked Questions (FAQs)

1. **Whether BCG can be reconstituted with distilled water, if diulent is not available?**

   No. Only the diluent supplied with the vaccine (0.9% sodium chloride) should be used. If not available, sterile *normal saline* may be used.

2. **Why local cleaning with spirit is not advised before BCG vaccination?**

   Site should be cleaned only with a sterile cotton swab and not with spirit or alcohol, which may affect the viability of bacilli in this live vaccine.

3. **Why is a lesser dose (0.05 ml) used under NIS in newborns <1 month?**

   Skin of the newborns is thin and large intradermal dose of 0.1 ml may break the skin or penetrate into deeper tissues, leading to infection. Dose of 0.05 ml is sufficient to elicit adequate protection. In fact, WHO and most manufacturers recommend smaller 0.05 ml dose till 1 year of age.

4. **Whether BCG can be given to Preterm and Low birth Weight infants?**

   BCG is safe and effective in healthy preterms above 32

weeks of gestation and probably also in LBW babies over 1500 gm. Data regarding efficacy of BCG in preterm <32 weeks or very low birth weight >1500 gm is limited and these cases may be vaccinated on discharge or follow-up.

5. **Why is it mandatory to give BCG intradermally? How can we ascertain that it has been given appropriately?**

BCG contains live attenuated bacilli, which multiply at the site of vaccination to provide sustained antigenic load. Subcutaneous or intramuscular injection leads to rapid clearance of bacilli via lymphatics affecting development of appropriate immune response. It is also associated with higher risk of BCG adenitis. A proper intra-dermal BCG injection should raise a wheal of ~5 mm over injection site, lasting for 15-30 min.

6. **A 7-year old child is being relocated from USA to India. Whether he needs BCG vaccination?**

BCG beyond 5 years is not generally recommended in India due to strong likelihood of natural infection by this age. However, this child coming from a low-risk country must receive BCG after TST, if negative and going to stay here for long time.

WHO recommends BCG to unvaccinated TST/IGRA negative older children and adults - a) residing in or moving to settings with high incidence of Tuberculosis and/or Leprosy or b) at risk of occupational exposure e.g. healthcare workers.

7. **What is accelerated BCG reaction?**

Some children, specially older ones, may develop induration at BCG site within 48–96 hours of vaccination rather than after 2-3 weeks (accelerated response), suggestive of previous exposure to tubercular infection. In the past, this accelerated response was used as an alternative to tuberculin test for presumptive diagnosis of infection (BCG Test), though no longer a valid test now.

8. **How can one assess the successful uptake of BCG vaccine?**

Successful uptake of BCG vaccine may be judged after 8–12 weeks, by - a) local scar formation, b) tuberculin conversion, or c) specific tests for cell-mediated immunity, e.g. Phytohemagglutinin test, Lymphocyte migration inhibition test etc., though rarely needed. However, No test is foolproof.

9. **A 3 month old infant has not yet developed the BCG scar despite documented vaccination at birth? What is to be done?.**

Apart from technical issues like use of wrong technique or heat-exposed vaccine, about 10% of BCG vaccinees do not develop scar and absence of scar does not necessarily mean vaccine failure. However in case of doubt, BCG may be repeated after 6 month of age on the opposite side, but only once. No tuberculin testing is required before revaccination in children below 5 years. There is no need to revaccinate the child beyond 5 years even if there is no scar due to high probability of natural infection. BCG scar may also disappear after 5–10 years of vaccination and does not indicate waning of immunity.

10. **What are the reasons for variations in reported efficacy of BCG?**

Suggested reasons for variably efficacy of BCG are - a) genetic variation in BCG strains. B) genetic variation in populations, c) background exposure rate - pre-vaccination exposure with natural disease may dampen the protective value of BCG in high-TB load populations, d) Interference by non-tuberculous mycobacteria leading to development of a non-specific immune response that masks further augmentation of the response following BCG vaccination, e) Interference by concurrent parasitic infection, which may produce a simultaneous Th2 response, blunting the Th1 response to BCG.

11. **A 2-month old BCG vaccinated infant at birth developed a non-healing ulcer at the injection site with painless axillary lymphadenopathy of ~1 cm on same side. How should it be managed?**

Following BCG vaccination, an indurated papule of 4-8 mm develops at the site after 2-3 weeks, which may ulcerates by 6-8 weeks and get covered with a crust, before forming a tiny round scar of 2-10 mm by 6-12 weeks. Some papules do not ulcerate at all, while other may ulcerate many times, before eventual scarring. A small (<1.5 cm) non-adherent ipsilateral lymph-node enlargement is also common during this period and No intervention is indicated in this case.

12. **Axillary Lymphadenopathy in abovementioned case was found to be AFB positive on Fine needle aspiration done elsewhere. Whether he needs antitubecular therapy?**

BCG lymphadenitis may be positive for acid-fast bacilli due to presence of bovine vaccine bacilli and should not be misconstrued as suggestive of tubercular disease. Antitubercular therapy is not indicated.

13. **How to treat regional BCG Lymphadenopathy?**

BCG lymphadenitis may be either *non-suppurative* or *suppurative* with development of fluctuation and erythema.

No treatment is required for *non-suppurative lymphadenitis*, which usually regress spontaneously in few weeks or months. Surgical drainage should be avoided to prevent sinus formation. Antibiotics or antitubercular therapy do not hasten the regression of nodes or prevent development of suppuration.

Suppurative lymphadenitis may perforate spontaneously with sinus formation and subsequent closure of the sinus by cicatrization. Fine needle aspiration or surgical excision of these nodes may be indicated, along with antibiotics to hasten resolution and prevent sinus formation.

Antitubercular therapy is indicated only in cases with rapidly progressive regional lymphadenitis, followed by removal of large nodes, if necessary, after completion of therapy.

14. What are the risk-factors for BCG lymphadenitis?

While it is difficult to predict possible risk factors for BCG lymphadenitis, commonly implicated ones include - a) higher dose, b) faulty administration, c) vaccination in neonatal period, d) immunodeficiency states and e) use of a vaccine with higher residual virulence of strain or higher viability (the proportion of living and dead bacilli). *Danish strain*, commonly used in India, is considered as more reactogenic.

15. Whether BCG can be given to a child born to mother with tuberculosis, along with INH prophylaxis.

While INH prophylaxis in a baby may affect viability of live bacilli in the vaccine theoretically, it has not been documented in practice and it is better to vaccinate even if the efficacy is doubtful.

However, WHO recommends that asymptomatic neonates born to mothers with bacteriologically confirmed pulmonary tuberculosis should be vaccinated at the end of preventive treatment, provided they are asymptomatic, HIV negative and have no immunological evidence of tubercular infection.

16. Whether BCG can be given to a baby borne to HIV infected mother?

HIV-infected newborns when vaccinated with BCG at birth are at higher risk of developing disseminated disease. However, considering benefits, WHO recommends that -

- Neonates born to women of unknown HIV status should be vaccinated at birth as the benefits outweigh the risks.

- Perinatally exposed neonates with unknown-HIV status born to HIV-infected women should be vaccinated, if there is no clinical evidence of HIV infection, regardless of whether the mother is receiving ART. (Note: Since BCG is given at birth when HIV status of newborn is unknown, practically all newborns, even if born to HIV-infected mothers must receive BCG)

- Children with confirmed HIV-infection and on antiretroviral therapy, should also be vaccinated with BCG, If not received at birth, if they are clinically well and immunologically stable with CD4 count > 25% for children below 5 years.

NACO Guidelines 2018 recommend that HIV exposed infants, like all other infants, should be given BCG at birth. However, If not given at birth, it should not be given in symptomatic HIV-infected older infants and children. IAP recommends BCG vaccination to all HIV infected children at birth, if they are asymptomatic.

17. What are the other uses of BCG vaccines?

BCG has also shown to be effective in preventing leprosy (RR 20-80%) and Buruli ulcer (RR 50%) in Africa. BCG is also used in high doses as immunotherapy in treatment of bladder cancers, given intravesically.

18. What is the status of newer anti-TB vaccines?

BCG is the only vaccine available against Tuberculosis, which is already a century old (developed in 1921) and being used despite questionable efficacy due to lack of alternatives. However, several new anti-tuberculosis vaccines are under development, some to boost pre-existing immunity induced by BCG and others to replace BCG as the primary vaccine. These vaccines target prevention of infection in naïve individuals *or* prevention of reactivation of latent infection *or* therapeutic vaccines to prevent relapses in TB patients. Currently, most favored research includes development of recombinant modified BCG vaccines, attenuated strains of Mycobacterium tuberculosis, subunit vaccines and DNA vaccines.

Key Points

- **Vaccine**: Live attenuated vaccine

- **Dose**: ID 0.05 ml over left shoulder (1.0 ml after 1 mo of age)

- **Schedule**: At birth or at first contact, may be clubbed with other vaccines at 6 weeks of age

- **Catch-up immunization**: Upto 5 years (one year in NIS)

- **Efficacy**: Controversial. ~70-90% for severe disease, ~50-60% for Pulm TB

- **Safety**: Regional Lymphadenitis, Disseminated disease

- **Contraindications**: Immunodeficiency states

References

1. World Health Organization. BCG vaccines: Position paper. Wkly Epidemiol Rec. 2018;93:73-96.
2. Parthasarthy A et al. Questions pertaining to Bacillus Calmette Guerin Vaccine. *In:* Vashishtha V et al. FAQs on Vaccines and immunization practices. 2nd Edition. New Delhi, Jaypee Brothers 2015; pp 99-106.
3. Shivanananda S. Bacillus Calmette Guerin Vaccine. *In:* IAP Guidebook on Immunization 2018-19 - Advisory Committee on Vaccines and Immunization

Practices, Indian Academy of Pediatrics, 3rd Edition, New Delhi, Jaypee Brothers 2020; pp 93-101.

4. Mangtani P et al. Protection by BCG vaccine against tuberculosis: A systematic review of randomized controlled trials. Clin Infect Dis. 2014;58 (4):470-80.

5. Ministry of Health and Family welfare, Government of India. National Immunization Schedule and Frequently asked questions In: Immunization Handbook for health workers 2018; pp 17-26.

6. Roy et al. Effect of BCG vaccination against Mycobacterium tuberculosis infection in children: systematic review and meta-analysis. BMJ 2014; Aug 5: 349:g4643.

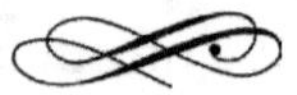

Hepatitis B Vaccine

Hepatitis B virus (HBV) is a leading cause of chronic liver disease and hepatocellular carcinoma in later life. Currently, 3-4% of Indian population is chronic HBV carrier (HBsAg positive for over 6 months). While most infected cases are asymptomatic in childhood, as many as 25% die due to chronic liver disease as adults.

Epidemiology: HBV, also referred as *Dane particle*, is a DNA virus containing many antigens, including a surface antigen (*HbsAg*), a core antigen (*HbcAg*) and a non-structural antigen (*HbeAg*). HBeAg serves as a marker of active viral replication and usually correlates with HBV DNA levels. HBV genotypes A and D are prevalent in India.

Persons with chronic HBV infection are primary reservoir of infection. Infection in children is predominantly acquired vertically from infected mothers apart from occasional cases of horizontal transmission following transfusions or as sexual-transmitted infection.

In India, ~2.5-3.0% pregnant women are HBsAg positive with ~10-85% risk of transmission of infection to their newborns. Risk of perinatal transmission largely depends on the mother's HBeAg status and 70-90% of infants born to HBeAg positive mothers becoming chronic carriers. Multiple blood transfusions is second commonest cause of HBV infections in children. Risk of becoming chronic carrier is higher in children infected at younger age.

Vaccine: Currently available HBV vaccines are all recombinant vaccines, containing the surface antigen of hepatitis B

(HbSAg), adjuvanted with aluminium salts and preserved with thiomerosal. Thiomerosal-free vaccines are also available.

Contents & storage: HBV vaccines are generally available as single-dose vials or prefilled syringes, containing Pediatric dose (10 µg/0.5 ml) or adult dose (20 µg/ml). Multi-dose vials and Combination vaccines as DPT + HBV ± HIB ± IPV and HAV + HBV are also available.

HBV Vaccine is relatively heat stable, though should be stored on 2–8°C. It should not be frozen and must be discarded, if frozen accidentally.

Dosage & administration: Pediatric dose ((10 µg/0.5 ml) is used till 18 years of age, given intramuscularly over deltoid or anterolateral thigh region. Gluteal injections should be avoided due to lower immunogenicity. Adult dose (20 µg/ml) is needed in older cases >18 years.

Immunization Schedule: In NIS, total four doses are given, one at birth (preferably within 24 hours) as a stand-alone vaccine, followed by three doses at 6,10 and 14 weeks of age as combination Pentavalent vaccine (DPT+HBV+HIB).

IAP concurs with NIS but suggests that last HBV dose should be administered not earlier than 24 weeks of age and at least 16 weeks after the first dose, whichever is later.

HBV schedules for infant immunization are widely flexible with minimum 3 doses at minimum 1 month interval, though preferred schedule is 0, 1, 6 months. Other acceptable alternatives are 0, 6, 14 weeks or 6, 10, 14 weeks.

Catch-up immunization is recommended, irrespective of the age, with three-dose schedule as 0, 1, 6 month. Pre-vaccination antibody screening is not recommended except in contacts of an HBsAg positive case. Under NIS, Catch-up HBV is given only till 1 year of age.

No booster is required except in cases with antibody titers below protective level (<10 mIU/ml), though post-vaccination antibody screening after 1 month of the last dose is recommended only in children born to HBsAg positive mothers, health workers and those with co-morbidities. Non-responders should be tested for HBV carrier status and if negative, must be revaccinated with same three-dose schedule. Almost all respond to revaccination and no further testing or revaccination is needed.

Efficacy of HBV relates to the induction of anti-HBs antibodies and memory T-cells. An anti-HBs concentration of 10 mIU/ml, 1–3 months after last dose is considered a reliable correlate of protection.

Three-dose vaccine series induces protective antibody concentrations in > 95% of healthy vaccinees and provides long-lasting immunity for up to 20 years or more though antibody titers may decline overtime. Periodic antibody testing is recommended only in children born to HBsAg positive mothers, health-care workers and those with co-morbidities.

HBV is a T-cell dependent vaccine and the titers at the end of immunization schedule may not be important as long as above the protective level. An anamnestic response will ensure adequate protection on re-exposure to the virus.

Safety: Side-effects are rare, except local pain, erythema and transient fever in some cases. HBV vaccines do not interfere with the immune response to other vaccines and vice versa.

Contraindications are none, except in rare instances of serious allergic reactions to previous dose.

Frequently Asked Questions (FAQs)

1. **Why is the *"birth dose"* of HBV vaccinee given within 24 hours of birth?**

    HBV is known to reduce the risk of perinatal HBV transmission by 18-40% only if given within the first 24 hours. Any dose given after 24 hours is not effective and hence not considered as *birth dose*.

2. **Why should an infant receive HBV vaccine at birth or before hospital discharge, even if mother is not HBsAg positive?**

    Since HBV status of mother may not be known at birth or there may be errors in testing, *Birth dose* of HBV acts as a safety net to prevent perinatal transmission in newborns in such cases. Delayed administration of the first dose beyond 7th day of life has been shown to increase rates of HBsAg acquisition in later life.

3. **Whether HBV Birth dose can be given to preterm and LBW infants?**

    Immunological response may be poor in preterms weighing <2000 gm and the vaccination strategy in them differs according to mother's HBsAg status. In these cases (Preterms <2000 gms) with -

    *   *HbsAg Negative mothers*, birth must be deferred till chronological age of 1 month.

    *   *HBsAg positive mothers*, birth dose must be given (along with HBIG) but not counted, to be followed by three subsequent doses at usual time. In these babies, HBsAg and Anti-HBsAg titers must be checked one month after the last dose to ensure effective immunization or transmission of infection. While anti-HBsAg is present in both, anti-HBcAg is positive only in natural infection.

4. **What should be the HBV schedule for an infant who missed the birth dose?**

Infants who miss the birth dose should receive three doses as soon as feasible with minimum interval of 4 weeks between first and second dose, and 8 weeks between second and third dose. Third dose should preferably be given not before 24 weeks of age or 16 weeks of last dose, whichever is later.

5. **Why HBV vaccine is given only upto 1 yr of age in UIP?**

In NIS, HBV is given only till one year of age as infections acquired in the first year of life have 90% chance of becoming chronic as compared to 30% during 1–5 years and 6% after 5 years. However, IAP recommends catch-up immunization in all older healthy children or adults with three-doses at 0, 1, 6 month schedule without pre-vaccination antibody screening (except in contacts of a HBsAg positive case).

6. **Whether HBV Vaccine can be used in Immunocom-promised cases?**

Yes. However, seroconversion rates are lower in the elderly, immunocompromised cases or in cases with chronic renal failure. In them, four doses at 0, 1, 2 and 12 months of *double dose* of vaccine may be given.

7. **Whether HBV boosters are required?**

No, except when antibody titers fall below protective level (<10 mIU/ml). However, periodic antibody testing is recommended only in infants born to HBsAg positive mothers or high-risk health-care workers. In those with titers below the protective levels (and not HBV carrier) same three-dose schedule should be repeated. Almost all respond to re-vaccination.

8. **A child vaccinated with four dose of HBV as per NIS schedule (0, 6, 10, 14 weeks) received an additional dose at 6 months by oversight (IAP recommendation) or at 18 months, due to use of a combination vaccine.**

    No. There is no harm or benefit of extra dose of HBV.

9. **Whether HBV vaccine can be used for Pre-exposure prophylaxis and How?**

    Pre-exposure prophylaxis is recommended to all health-care and laboratory personnel with three doses of HBV vaccine at 0, 1, 6 months (If required, an accelerated schedule may be used at 0, 4, 12 weeks). Vaccinees with direct patient contact or handling blood specimens should also have post-vaccination testing for anti-HBS antibodies after one month of the last dose to identify non-responders who need re-vaccination. No further periodic testing or booster doses are required in immu-nocompetent vaccinees.

10. **What should be done to prevent perinatal transmission of infection in newborns of HBsAg positive mothers?**

    All Infants born to HbsAg positive mothers should receive both, HBV vaccine as well as HBIG (IM 0.5 ml each) as early as possible, preferably within 12 hours of birth at two different sites. It should be followed by regular HBV vaccination at 6, 10 and 14 weeks. Although HBIG may be given up to 7 days of birth, if not available earlier, efficacy after 48 hours is not known. Breast feeding is not contraindicated by HBsAg positive mother, if she is HBeAg negative, and does not increase the risk of transmission.

    All infants born to positive mothers should be tested for HBsAg and anti-HBsAg antibodies at 9–15 months to identify carriers (HBsAg+ve) or non-responders (anti-HBsAg -ve). Re-vaccination is required only if both markers are negative (non-carrier/non-responder).

11. **What should be done to prevent perinatal transmission in newborns of mothers with unknown HBsAg status?**

All Infants born to mothers with unknown HBsAg status, should receive HBV within 12 hours of birth and mother's status should be checked as early as possible. HBIG must be administered to all babies after maternal status is known and positive, which should not be delayed beyond 12 hours of birth in babies < 2000 gm and 7 days in heavier babies.

12. **Whether HBV vaccine alone can be used for perinatal prophylaxis to newborns of HbSAg positive mothers, if HBIG is not available or unaffordable.**

HBV along may be given at 0, 1 and 2 months with an additional dose between 9 and 12 months, if HBIG is not available or unaffordable. However, the efficacy of perinatal prophylaxis with both HBIG and HBV is 85–95% as compared to 70-75% with HBV-birth dose alone.

13. **What is the Post-exposure prophylaxis against high-risk HBV exposure e.g. needle stick injury or infected blood transfusion?**

HBV can survive in dried blood or on contaminated surfaces for at least one week and the risk of transmission to exposed persons depends on - a) degree of contact, b) HBeAg status of the source person, and c) HBV vaccination status of the exposed. All high-risk exposures following needle-stick injury, infected blood transfusion or contact of mucous membrane/ non-intact skin with potentially infectious body fluids must receive post-exposure prophylaxis as follows (**Table 8.1**)-

- All exposures to a source with unknown HBsAg status should be considered as positive exposures. However, the source should be tested for HBsAg status as early as possible.

Table 8.1: Post-exposure prophylaxis for HBV			
Exposed *(Check HBV vaccination status & Assess Anti HbSAg titers after one month)*		**Source** *(Test for HbSAg as soon as possible)*	
Vaccination Status*	**Anti HbS titers#**	**HbSAg Positive/ unknown$**	**Negative**
No	–	HBIG+HBV	HBV
Yes	Protective	No Rx	No Rx
Yes	Non-protective (Revaccinate)	HBIG%+HBV	HBV
Yes	Unknown	HBIG+HBV	HBV

*Three or more HBV doses, # > 10 mIU/ml, $ test as early as possible
% exposed persons with non-protective serotiters despite 6 doses of HBV 'should receive 2nd dose of HBIG one month after first dose'.

- No intervention is needed, if *exposed person* is - a) fully vaccinated with known protective titers, b) known chronic carrier or c) had HBV infection in the past.

- No intervention is needed if the *source* is known HBsAg negative, though opportunity must be used to give/complete HBV vaccination.

- All other exposures must receive HBIG and first dose of HBV vaccine, as early as possible, at different sites and complete HBV vaccination with two further doses (0, 1, 6 mo).

- Test anti-HBsAg titers after 1 month of last dose and revaccinate once again with 3 doses (0, 1, 6 mo), if not protective (<10 mIU/ml).

- Recipients of infected blood transfusions must be tested again after 1 year for HBsAg as well as anti-HbsAg titers. While HBsAg positivity suggests chronic infection, simultaneous presence of anti HBsAg antibodies indicates lesser risk of infectivity.

14. What is the role of Hepatitis B Immunoglobulin (HBIG) in HBV prevention?

HBIG is indicated to provide short-term passive immunity (3-6 mo) along with HBV in perinatally exposed newborns or horizontally exposed susceptible individuals, given as 0.5 ml intramuscularly in infants (0.06 ml/kg IM in older children or adults). HBIG is also used alone for post-exposure prophylaxis in persons who are non-responders to HBV (Genetic/ immunocompromised) with two doses at one month interval. *It should not be given Intravenously.* Few IV preparations (Hepatect CP®) are available, but with uncertain efficacy.

Key Points

- **Vaccine:** Recombinant, available as stand-alone or combination Vaccine

- **Dose:** IM 0.5 ml/dose (1 ml >18 yrs age) over thigh/deltoid

- **Schedule:**

  - NIS: Total 4 doses at birth, 6, 10 & 14 weeks, No boosters

  - IAP: Total 4 doses at birth, 6, 10 weeks & 6 months
    (Last dose not before 24 wk of age or 16 wk of first dose)

- **Catch-up immunization:** 0, 1, 6 mo, No upper age limit (upto 1 yr in NIS)

- **Efficacy** >95% for at least 20 years

- **Safety:** Side-effects rare, except Local reaction or mild fever

- **Contraindications:** None except hypersensitivity to previous dose

---

References

1. World Health Organization. Hepatitis B vaccines: Position paper. Weekly Epid. Record 2017;92:369-392)

2. Kalra A et al. Hepatitis B vaccine. *In:* Vashishtha V et al. FAQs on Vaccines

and immunization practices. 2nd Edition. .New Delhi, Jaypee Brothers 2015; pp 99-106.

3. Shivanananda S. Hepatitis B vaccine. *In:* IAP Guidebook on Immunization 2018-19 - Advisory Committee on Vaccines and Immunization Practices, Indian Academy of Pediatrics, 3rd Edition, New Delhi, Jaypee Brothers 2020; pp 122-131.

4. Ministry of Health and Family welfare, Government of India. National Immunization Schedule and Frequently asked questions *In:* Immunization Handbook for health workers 2018; pp 17-26.

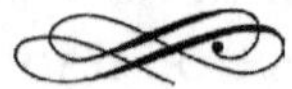

Polio Vaccines

After successful eradication of smallpox, Poliomyelitis is the second vaccine preventable disease on the verge of eradication following WHO's *global polio eradication initiative*, launched in 1988. In 2021 (till May), only two cases of wild polio virus (WPV) disease have been reported from two countries - one each from Pakistan and Afghanistan, as compared to 140 cases in 2020, all from these two countries.

Epidemiology: Poliovirus is a small RNA enterovirus with three serotypes—Types 1, 2 and 3, also known as *Brunhilde, Lancing* and *Leon* respectively. Infection is generally transmitted feco-orally from a symptomatic or carrier case excreting virus in stools. Contaminated water supply and poor immunization coverage are two important determinants of polio transmission. Since the virus cannot survive outside human body for long, prime strategy of polio eradication revolves around expanding immunization coverage to minimize the availability of susceptible hosts for virus infection and transmission.

Out of the three WPV serotypes, two have been declared eradicated globally –Type 2 in 2015 and Type 3 in October 2019. Currently, all reported cases are due to type 1 serotype. In India, No Poliomyelitis case has been reported since 13th January 2011 and WHO has declared India polio-free w.e.f. 27th March 2014.

Vaccines: Two types of polio vaccines are available - an inactivated, parenteral *Salk vaccine (IPV)* and another live, oral, *Sabin vaccine (OPV)*. Till 2017, only OPV was used under NIS in India and IPV has been added subsequently for the final assault against disease.

9.1: ORAL POLIO VACCINE

Developed by Albert Sabin (1961) OPV vaccine is presently available as *Bivalent* (bOPV) containing serotype 1 & 3 (BioPolio® B1/3, Others). Trivalent OPV including all three serotypes has been discontinued since August 2016 after eradication of type 2 disease. A monovalent type 2 vaccine (mOPV2) has been kept for stockpiling in case of post-eradication outbreaks.

Contents & Storage: Currently available OPV is a *live attenuated, bivalent* vaccine (bOPV), containing serotype 1 and 3, in concentrations of 10^6 and $10^{5.8}$ CCID50, respectively. Some brands contain Phenol red as indicator to give it a light pink color.

OPV is supplied as multi-dose vials with dropper. It is extremely heat-sensitive and maintenance of adequate cold chain is essential with depot level storage at -18 to -20°C till expiry and peripheral centers storage at 2-8°C for 6 months. Multiple freeze-thaw cycles should be avoided as the virus loses its potency. It must reach immunization center at 2–8°C in vaccine carriers. Each OPV vial is also marked with vaccine vial monitor.

Dosage & administration: OPV is given as 2 drops orally. It is preferable, though not necessary, to defer breastfeeding for about 15-30 minutes after administration.

Immunization Schedule: *NIS* includes total six doses of OPV as one at birth *(Zero dose)*, three primary doses at 6,10 and 14 weeks and a booster dose at 16-24 months *(along with* two doses of fractionated IPV at 6 and 14 weeks, discussed later). Additional doses of OPV given during pulse polio campaign should not be counted for routine immunization purpose.

IAP recommend only one dose of OPV at birth (zero dose) for routine immunization, with replacement of subsequent doses by IM-IPV (6,10,14 weeks and two Boosters at 16-18 months and 4-6 years, discussed later). However, additional doses of OPV under pulse polio campaign should continue. IAP also recommends that *no child should be immunized with bOPV alone* and if availability or affordability of IPV is an issue, s/he may be given a combination vaccine containing IPV or must be referred to a government healthcare facility for the primary immunization as per UIP schedule.

Efficacy: Protective efficacy of OPV depends on the development of humoral immunity (circulating neutralizing antibody) and mucosal immunity (secretory IgA).

Presence of neutralizing antibody against polioviruses is considered a reliable correlate of immunogenicity. While tOPV was nearly 100% immunogenic in developed countries, data from developing countries including India, suggested a lower seroconversion rates after three doses i.e. ~65% for type 1 and 3 and ~95% for type 2 serotype. Poor immunogenicity in developing countries was thought to be due to interference of maternal antibodies with early primary doses, poor intestinal immunity in malnourished or zinc-deficient children and presence of diarrhea or other enteric infections at the time of vaccination etc.

tOPV to bOPV shift: Bivalent OPV is considered as more immunogenic than trivalent OPV, as competition between different viral strains for mucosal uptake is reduced. In trivalent OPV, type 2 strain was taken preferentially and interfered with immunological responses to other serotypes. World, as well as India, has switched over from tOPV to bOPV (without type 2 strain following its eradication from 2015).

After a trivalent or bivalent OPV dose, uptake is competitive and all serotypes of the vaccine might not be able to attach with receptor sites in the gut. Hence, multiple doses are necessary for primary immunization to ensure uptake of all serotypes. Efficacy of the OPV known to increase from 80 to 90% after 3 and 5 doses respectively.

Birth-dose: Studies from India demonstrated that the infants who receive a birth dose of OPV achieve higher levels of neutralizing antibodies and seroconversion rates following subsequent OPV/IPV doses in early infancy. Moreover, OPV at birth can induce mucosal protection before enteric pathogens interfere with the immune response, and prevent VAPP.

Mucosal immunity in polio refers to the resistance against mucosal infection by wild virus due to prior infection with vaccine viruses. Mucosal immunity decreases the replication and shedding of the virus, and provides a potential barrier to its transmission. OPV has to advantage of providing better mucosal immunity than the IPV, though it tends to wane over time and repeated doses are necessary to maintain sufficient mucosal immunity. No definite data is available from developing countries about the duration of mucosal immunity for polioviruses. However, even fully immunized older children are known to have WPV1 infection and fecal shedding when come in contact with under-5 children with polio, perhaps due to high viral load of wild infection inoculums.

Herd effect refers to the phenomenon of reduced disease load *even in unimmunized population* following good immunization coverage of the susceptible population, due to reduced opportunities for the transmission of the disease. Higher is the vaccine efficacy and coverage, greater is the herd effect. After an OPV dose, vaccinia virus is excreted in stools for variable period. Ability of the OPV to infect contacts of vaccine recipients (*Contact immunity*) due to transient viral shedding from gut and upper respiratory tract after 4-6 weeks of vaccination is considered as an important advantage of OPV compared with IPV to minimize transmission of wild virus (Herd effect). OPV provides good herd immunity in industrialized countries, though such robust herd effect has not been visible in India.

Safety: OPV is extremely safe, except potential but very rare risk of vaccine-related disease i.e. *Vaccine associated Paralytic polio* (VAPP) and *vaccine derived Polio virus* (VDPV). These cases were more common with tOPV use and Risk has been nearly halved after switch-over to bOPV due to elimination of type 2 virus.

Vaccine associated paralytic polio *(VAPP)* is an extreme rare complication (1:4 million doses), more common with first dose (1:3 million doses) then subsequent-doses (1:13.9 million). Perhaps, the first dose provides some immunity before subsequent doses to prevent VAPP.

VAPP risk is relatively lower in India than in developed countries due to presence of maternal antibodies, birth dose of OPV and lower "take-up" of the vaccine (only the vaccine that is taken up, can cause VAPP).

Clinically defined as *acute flaccid paralysis with residual weakness for 60 days after the onset of symptoms and isolation of vaccine virus in stools*, VAPP is caused by loss of attenuating mutations during replication of the virus in the gut, reverting its neurovirulence.

VAPP may develop in a vaccine recipient within 4-40 days of receiving OPV *(recipient VAPP)* or in unimmunized contact of the vaccine recipient, who is shedding virus in stools *(contact VAPP)*. However, virus does not spread beyond close contacts and there are no VAPP outbreaks.

Majority of recipient VAPP cases are associated with type 3 virus (42%), followed by type 2 (26%), type 1 (20%), and mixed (15%).

Vaccine derived polioviruses *(VDPV)* denotes mutation of parent vaccine virus with >1% divergence from the original strain (>0.6% for type 2). These mutant viruses are not only neurovirulent, but also transmissible and capable of causing outbreaks. VDPV is more common following vaccination of immunodeficient children.

VDPV are classified as – a) *cVDPV* with evidence of virus circulation in the population, b) *iVDPV* in the immunodeficient person, and c) *aVDPV* of ambiguous origin isolated from environment or from an immunocompetent person with no evidence of circulation.

cVDPV, the commonest cause of vaccine-virus associated outbreaks, is defined as genetically linked VDPVs isolated from – a) at least two individuals, not necessarily AFP cases, who are not household contacts, b) one individual and one or more environmental surveillance samples, or c) at least two environmental samples from different collection sites without overlapping of catchment areas, or from one site at interval of > 2 months.

About 90% of reported cVDPV are due to type 2 virus and risk factors for cVDPV outbreaks include – a) drop in OPV coverage , b) elimination of the corresponding WPV serotype and c) poor AFP surveillance to detect circulating mutant virus. Continuation of cVDPV circulation in the population for more than six months is denoted as *persistent cVDPV*. Outbreaks have the ability to become endemic and spread to other under-vaccinated communities and countries. cVDPVs can be stopped with 2 to 3 rounds of high-quality, large-scale supplementary immunization activities. Risk of VDPVs is the reason why synchronous stopping of tOPV use globally and continuing to vaccinate with IPV is mandatory in the post-polio eradication scenario.

Possibility of VAPP/VDPV should be considered in any case of acute flaccid paralysis with history of – a) OPV vaccination in preceding 30 days, b) Contact with recently immunized child in preceding 60 days, or c) Mass immunization program, i.e. *pulse polio* in the community, in preceding 60 days. **Table 9.1** provides important difference between VAPP

Table 9.1: VAPP vs cVDPV		
Difference	**VAPP**	**cVDPV**
Caused by..	Loss of attenuation in vaccine virus	Mutation in parent virus
Commonest strain	PV 3 (42%)	PV2 (90%)
Occurs in..	Vaccine recipients & close contacts	Any under-immunized Child
Timing	Within 60 days of vaccination/contact	Any time
Clustering	Usually isolated case	May be in clusters/ Outbreaks
Risk of spread	Negligible	High

and cVDPV, though final differentiation is possible only on virological studies.

Contraindications are none except a child with immunodeficiency disorder in self or any other house-hold member to avoid risk of iVDPV. HIV infection does not appear to be a risk factor for VAPP.

9.2: INJECTABLE (SALK) POLIO VACCINE (IPV)

IPV vaccine developed by Dr Jonas Salk , though licensed since 1955, was out of favour for many decades due to ease of administration and advantage of better local immunity with OPV. However, considering the potential risk of VAPP/ VDPV with OPV, specially as the world nears the eradication phase of disease, led to re-introduction of IPV in immunization schedules of many countries. In India, IPV was licensed in 2006 and has been introduced in NIS since 2016-17.

Contents & Storage: IPV is a Trivalent vaccine, containing formaldehyde-inactivated 40, 8 and 32 D antigen units of poliovirus type 1, 2 and 3 respectively from selected strains. All currently available IPV are also *enhanced potency* or eIPV, containing 40 D Antigen units of WPV1 versus 20 D units in older products.

IPV is available as multi-dose vial under national program and as single dose (0.5 ml) vial/pre-filled syringe for commercial use (Poliovac®, Imovax Polio®, polprotec®). IPV is also available as hexavalent vaccine in combination with Pentavalent Vaccines for primary immunization (Easysix®, Hexaxim®, Infanrix-Hexa®) and with DTaP/TdaP vaccines (Tetraxim®) for booster doses.

IPV should be stored at 2–8°C. Multi-dose vials can be used up to 28 days after opening, under open vial policy.

Dosage & administration: Regular IPV dose is 0.5 ml intramuscularly/subcutaneously given over lateral aspect of the thigh. However in NIS, 1/5th fraction of this dose (fIPV) i.e. 0.1 ml is given Intradermally.

Immunization Schedule: NIS uses *combined OPV-IPV schedule* with two doses of fIPV at 6th and 14th week, along with five doses of OPV at birth, 6-10-14 weeks and 16-24 months. (No *IPV* at birth, 10 weeks or Booster). Under NIS, IPV is given only till 1 year of age.

IAP recommend total five doses of IPV – Three primary doses at 6,10 and 14 weeks, and two booster doses at 16-18 month and 4-6 years, along with *only one* dose of OPV at birth. Stand-alone or Combination vaccines including IPV can be used for these doses. Additional doses of OPV under pulse polio campaign should continue.

Catch-up immunization is recommended to children < 5 years of age who have completed primary immunization with OPV alone, with three doses at 0, 2 and 6 months, to ensure long-lasting protection.

Efficacy: IPV is highly immunogenic, depending on age of vaccination, number of doses and interval between doses. Immune response is dampened by the presence of maternal antibodies in the very young infant <6-8 weeks. Seroconversion rates with three IM-IPV doses at 6, 10 and 14 weeks is reported to be ~ 85.8%, 86.2%, and 96.9% for serotypes 1, 2, and 3. Even with two IM-IPV doses at two months interval seroconversion rates are about ~ 89%, 92% and 70% for three serotypes respectively. Antibodies titers fall after primary doses but remain protective till the first booster in second year of life to produce strong anamnestic response, which ensures the perpetuation of immunity for decades. IPV as combination vaccine is equally effective. Immunological response to 3-dose IPV is satisfactory in preterm infants, though titers might be lower than in term infants, particularly if they are chronically ill.

Fractional doses of IPV, given intradermally, reduce the cost and allows immunization of larger number of children with limited vaccine supply. Although antibody titers after two doses of fIPV are lower than two conventional IM-IPV doses, seroconversion rates are comparable, and better than one IM-IPV dose.

Mucosal immunity: IPV is less effective than OPV in inducing IgA mediated intestinal mucosal immunity, though it generates stronger humoral immunity. It has been postulated that the spill-over of IgG antibodies has inhibitory influence on local infection.

Birth-dose: Studies have shown that Infants who receive a birth dose of IPV (or within 2 weeks) have higher seroconversion rates with stronger antibody titers following primary doses than those who have not received it, similar to OPV. However, OPV is preferable as birth dose due to better mucosal protection before enteric pathogens interfere with the immune response.

Safety: IPV vaccines are safe except minor and transient local reactions e.g. erythema, induration, and tenderness. As IPV contains traces of streptomycin, neomycin and polymyxin B, hypersensitivity reactions to these antimicrobials are possible.

Contraindications are none except history of allergy to previous dose or the preservatives used in the vaccine. IPV can be used in immunodeficient children without risk of VDPV.

Frequently Asked Questions (FAQs)

1. **What is the need to continue Polio vaccination in India when it has been eliminated from the country?**

   WPV disease still occurs in two countries – Pakistan and Afganistan. Until the worldwide polio eradication is achieved, risk of imported WPV from endemic countries or cases due to circulating vaccine derived poliovirus (cVDPV), continues unless population immunity is maintained by universal immunization.

2. **What was the need to add IPV in immunization schedule when OPV has been largely successful?**

   OPV has worked fantastically to eliminate wild virus disease from country and India has been declared Polio-free since 27th March 2014. However, two important issues hamper further success with OPV alone – a) Risk of VAPP/VDPV, and b) Fear of accidental WPV2 outbreaks due to use of PV2- free bivalent OPV vaccine.

   Hence, WHO recommended inclusion of at least one dose of IPV in the vaccination schedule of countries using OPV in their NIS to - a) reduce the risk of VAPP, and b) induce an immunity base that could be rapidly boosted if there is an outbreak due to WPV2 (IPV is a trivalent vaccine, containing PV2). Inclusion of IPV may also boost both humoral and mucosal immunity against poliovirus WPV1 & 3 in previous OPV recipients.

3. **Then, why doesn't India shift to only IPV (no OPV) schedule?**

IPV is highly immunogenic and protective but it cannot completely replace OPV in immunization schedule at present due to following reasons –

- IPV is less effective than OPV to induce IgA mediated gut mucosal immunity, though it generates stronger humoral immunity and spill-over of these IgG antibodies has inhibitory influence on local infection.

- Birth dose of IPV is less effective than OPV due to presence of maternal antibodies, which predominantly hamper development of systemic immunity of IPV rather than mucosal immunity of OPV.

- Immunogenicity of IPV depends on the number of doses and IPV-alone schedules recommend IM-IPV either with three doses (at 6, 10 and 14 weeks) or at least two doses (at 2 and 4 months) for adequate immunogenic response, which is difficult to provide at present due to short-supply of the IPV till recently.

- OPV needs to continue in Pulse polio program due to continued risk of wild virus import from neighbouring countries to maintain herd immunity. Ability of OPV to infect contacts of vaccine recipients (i.e. contact spread) and "indirectly vaccinate" them is considered as an advantage vis a vis IPV.

WHO recommends that countries at high risk for importation of poliovirus, should use bOPV at birth or within 7 days, followed by three primary bOPV doses at 6, 10, 14 weeks along with either atleast one IM-IPV dose at/after 14 weeks or two fIPV at 6 and 14 weeks. Two fIPV doses are more immunogenic than single IM-IPV dose, as used in NIS.

4. **What is the rationale behind use of fIPV rather than IM-IPV in national program?**

   WHO recommended at least one dose of IPV in the NIS of countries using OPV to reduce the risk of VAPP and to induce an immunity base that could be rapidly boosted if there is an outbreak due to WPV2.

   India began with introduction of single dose IM-IPV for primary immunization but later switched to two dose ID-IPV at 6 and 14 weeks using only 0.1 ml i.e. 1/5th fraction of IM dose (fIPV) to reduce the cost without compromising the efficacy and immunize larger population with limited vaccine supply.

   Two fractional doses of ID-IPV provide seroconversion rates higher than one full IM dose and comparable to two full IM doses, though antibody titers might be lower than two full doses.

5. **Then, why private sector does not follow the same schedule and uses costly IPV-containing combination vaccines?**

   Till recently stand-alone IPV was not freely available in Indian market and hence it was difficult to follow NIS in practice, necessitating use of combination vaccines. Further, with limited patient volume, use of fractional IPV is not cost-effective to private practitioners. Combination vaccines also offer convenience of lesser pricks.

6. **What should be done if Stand-alone IPV is not available in private clinic?**

   No child should be immunized with bOPV alone and if availability or affordability of IPV is an issue, s/he may be given a combination vaccine containing IPV or referred to a government healthcare facility for primary immunization as per UIP schedule

7. **A 3 year old child has been immunized with all doses of OPV including birth dose and booster, but without any dose of IPV due to non-availability at that time? Whether he needs IPV now?**

   Infants and young children, born after the switch from tOPV to OPV (25 April, 2016), who have not received IPV in any schedule, should receive at least one dose of an IPV/IPV combination vaccine, intramuscularly, at the earliest opportunity.

8. **What is the need for *zero dose* of OPV at birth and Whether IPV can be used for this purpose?**

   Zero (Birth) OPV dose aims to provide local gut immunity in a baby who is still protected by maternal antibodies to minimize the risk of VAPP after subsequent OPV exposure. Though OPV at birth by itself is not immunogenic, it enhances seroconversion rates after subsequent primary OPV/IPV doses. While a single dose of IPV at birth has also been shown to prime the Immune system and improve seroconversion rates after primary OPV/IPV doses, it is not as effective as OPV to produce local gut immunity. Thus, the children who receive IPV at birth remain at higher risk to shed OPV in their feces and transmit VAPP.

9. **Why the VAPP is less common in India than in developed countries.**

   VAPP risk is lower in India than in developed countries (1:2.4 million) due to presence of maternal antibodies, birth dose of OPV and lower *"take-up"* of the vaccine. Only the vaccine that is taken up can cause VAPP.

10. **How can one differentiate between VAPP and cVDPV?**

    Although both cases present with acute flaccid paralysis and final differentiation is possible only on virological studies, important differences between VAPP and cVDPV have been shown in **Table 9.1** In brief -

VAPP denotes loss of attenuating mutation in the vaccine virus during replication in the gut of recipient and hence, affects only the recipient or close unimmunized contact. Most cases of VAPP are isolated cases with history of receiving OPV themselves or in contacts and outbreak is *unlikely*. Majority of these cases are due to type 3 virus (42%).

However, VDPV denotes significant mutation of the vaccine virus which is now not only neurovirulent but is also transmissible. Mutant Virus is isolated from two or more individuals or environmental surveillance samples often over long periods and may lead to outbreaks or endemic disease. Most cases of VDPV are caused by type 2 virus.

11. Which vaccine should be used in immunodeficient children?

OPV is contraindicated in immunodeficient children, predominantly due to higher risk of iVDPV. IPV can be used in them, though seroconversion rates or antibody titers may not be optimal in them.

12. What are the recommendations for travelers to Polio-endemic countries?

IAP has issued the following recommendations for travelers to polio-endemic countries or areas:

- Those who have previously received at least 3 doses of OPV/IPV should be offered a single dose of OPV/IPV before departure.

- Non-immunized individuals should complete a primary schedule of polio vaccine, using atleast three doses of either IPV or OPV.

- For frequent travelers to the polio-endemic areas but who stay only for brief periods, a one-time additional dose of OPV/IPV after primary series should be sufficient to prevent disease.

13. What are current WHO recommendations for OPV immunization?

WHO suggests that the choice of polio vaccination schedules during pre-eradication phase should rest on probabilities of wild poliovirus importation, with following main recommendations -

- In countries with high risk of feco-oral transmission, use of bOPV is essential as it induces higher levels of intestinal immunity than IPV.

- At least one dose of IPV should be included in NIS of countries using OPV, to reduce the risk of VAPP and to induce an immunity base that could be rapidly boosted if there is an outbreak due to WPV2.

- For endemic countries or countries at high risk for importation of poliovirus, bOPV at birth or within 7 days, should be followed by three primary bOPV doses at 6, 10, 14 weeks along with either at least one IM-IPV dose at 14 weeks or two fIPV at 6 and 14 weeks. Two fIPV doses are more immunogenic than single IM-IPV dose. To mitigate the risk of undetected transmission, WHO recommends that these countries should not switch to an *IPV-only* schedule.

- Countries with sustained high vaccination coverage (>90-95%) and very low risk of WPV importation may consider an *IPV-only* schedule.

- Countries with insufficient vaccination coverage, should continue SIAs until routine coverage improves or until the globally-coordinated withdrawal of OPV.

- Ultimately, the use of OPV has to stopped after eradication of disease though at least one dose of IPV needs to continue for at least 5 years after OPV cessation.

14. What is Pulse polio immunization?

Pulse polio immunization (PPI) is a mass OPV immunization campaign to supplement routine immunization as well as to facilitate development of herd immunity, conducted annually and simultaneously *(pulse)* throughout the country on pre-fixed dates (National/ subnational immunization days i.e. NID/SNID)

15. How does PPI helps to eliminate Poliomyelitis?

As the vaccine-virus is excreted in stools for 4–6 weeks, simultaneous OPV administration to a large population leads to extensive dissemination of vaccine virus in community, which competes with wild-virus for gut uptake. Since wild virus cannot survive in external involvement for long, it is expected to be flushed-out from community.

16. Who should be immunized under PPI campaign?

Target population for PPI is all children <5 years of age (including newborns), irrespective of their previous immunization status. OPV doses during PPI are additional and should not replace doses of regular immunization. There are no contraindications for PPI dose and it should be given irrespective of the interval with dose given/due under routine immunization schedule.

17. What is Mop-up immunization for Poliomyelitis?

Mop-up immunization is a part of *intensified PPI* with extensive house-to-house immunization campaign to target children < 5 years with two doses of OPV at 4-6 weeks interval. These campaigns are conducted in high-risk areas identified on AFP surveillance to eliminate last reservoirs of wild viruses, in other-wise good immunization coverage areas.

18. What is Acute flaccid paralysis (AFP) surveillance?

AFP surveillance is an integral part of Global Polio eradication initiative, defined as *"an operational strategy to detect all cases of wild virus disease and eliminate remaining foci of polio transmission".*

19. What is AFP?

AFP is defined as *"any illness presenting with acute onset of flaccid paralysis in a child <15 years, for which no obvious cause such as trauma or electrolyte imbalance is found or a person of any age, with clinical suspicion of polio"*. Generally, a flaccid paralysis of < 4 weeks is considered as acute.

20. Why is it necessary to investigate all cases of AFP, when objective of the AFP surveillance is to detect cases of poliomyelitis?

Since it is difficult to exclude poliomyelitis in a suspected case without detailed investigations, it is essential to investigate each case of AFP under AFP surveillance program, to ensure that all cases of paralytic poliomyelitis are detected, reported and investigated and no case is missed out.

21. What is vaccine vial monitor?

Each OPV vial (and some other heat sensitive vaccines as well) is marked with *vaccine vial monitor*, i.e. a sticker with a lighter square inside a darker circle (**Fig. 9.1**). *If the color of square is darker or matching the outer circle, vaccine is probably not potent and should be discarded.*

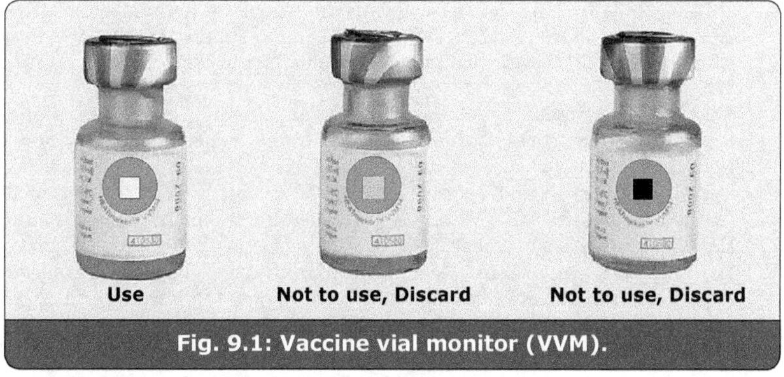

Fig. 9.1: Vaccine vial monitor (VVM).

Key points

Types: Live Oral (Sabin) & Inactivated Injectable (Salk) vaccine

Oral Polio vaccine (OPV)

- **Vaccine:** Live Attenuated, Bivalent (PV1 & 3), Liquid formulation
- **Dose:** PO 2 drops/dose
- **Schedule:**

  NIS: Total 5 doses: At Birth, 6,10,14 weeks, 16-24 mo

  IAP: Only one dose at Birth
- **Efficacy:** >95%, provides Local and Herd immunity
- **Safety:** Very rare risk of VAPP/VDPV
- **Contraindications:** Immunodeficiency disorders

Injectable Polio vaccine (IPV)

- **Vaccine:** Inactivated, Trivalent (PV1,2,3) Liquid formulation
- **Dose:** IM 0.5 ml/dose or ID 0.1ml/dose (Fractionated IPV)
- **Schedule:**

  NIS: Total 2 fractionated doses at 6 & 14 weeks

  IAP: Total 5 regular IM doses at 6, 10, 14 wks,15-18 mo and 5-6 yrs
- **Efficacy:** >95%, Spill-over mucosal immunity, Herd effect ?
- **Safety:** Local, Hypersensitivity
- **Contraindications:** H/O allergy to previous dose

References

1. World Health Organization, Polio vaccines. Position paper, Wkly Epidemiol Rec. 2016;91:145-168
2. Shivanananda S. Polio Vaccines. *In:* IAP Guidebook on Immunization 2018-19 - Advisory Committee on Vaccines and Immunization Practices, Indian Academy of Pediatrics, 3rd Edition, New Delhi, Jaypee Brothers 2020; pp 102-121.
3. Thacker N et al. Polio. *In:* Vashishtha V et al. FAQs on Vaccines and immunization practices. 2nd Edition. New Delhi, Jaypee Brothers 2015; pp 107-126.
4. Ministry of Health and Family welfare, Government of India. National Immunization Schedule and Frequently asked questions. In: Immunization Handbook for health workers 2018; pp 17-26.
5. World Health Organization Meeting of the Strategic Advisory Group of Experts on immunization, October 2017 conclusions and Recommendations on Polio vaccines. Wkly Epid. Record 2017;92:729-48.

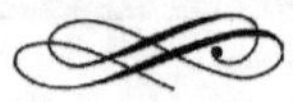

Vaccines against three common bacterial illnesses – Diphtheria, Pertussis (Whooping Cough) and Tetanus were earliest combination vaccines in use since 1940s, including Trivalent DPT, Bivalent DT and Monovalent TT.

Conventional DPT vaccine contains inactivated whole cell pertussis organisms, apart from Diphtheria toxoid and Tetanus toxoid, also referred as DTwP. Over time, this vaccine has been modified to - a) replace whole cell pertussis organisms with acellular bacterial antigens to minimize side-effects (DTaP), b) reduce the dose of diphtheria antigens to make it more suitable for use in older children and adolescents (Td or TdaP), and c) combine DTwP/DTaP with other antigens e.g. Hib, HBV and IPV to reduce the number of pricks.

Epidemiology

Diphtheria is an acute life-threatening illness, caused by three toxigenic strains (*gravis, intermidius and mitis*) of *C. diphtheria*– a gram positive bacilli, almost exclusively localized over respiratory mucosa of clinical cases or asymptomatic carriers. Infection is usually transmitted via droplets, fomites or rarely through direct contact with infected secretions. Disease is most common in pre-school unvaccinated children, during autumn and winter season. Infection is non-invasive and major virulence of organism lies in its ability to an *exotoxin,* responsible for local necrosis and systemic complications. All vaccines against Diphtheria use a toxoid i.e. inactivated toxin, as antigen.

Pertussis (Whooping cough) is a highly contagious respiratory infection due to *B. pertussis,* a gram-negative coccobacilli, present in nasopharyngeal secretions of clinical or sub-clinical case and spreads via droplets. Pertussis is primarily a disease of infants and toddlers, though can also occur in newborns due to negligible trans placental transfer of maternal antibodies and is being increasingly seen in older children due to shift in the age-epidemiology after expanding immunization coverage in infants. Maximum cases occur in late winter/early spring season. It is also largely a non-invasive infection with localised respiratory pathology, though a specific *pertussis toxin* and other bio-active substances, produced by the bacteria, contribute to pathology, clinical features and development of immunity. Vaccines against pertussis contain either the inactivated whole bacterial cell (wP) or selective antigens (aP).

Tetanus is also an acute life-threatening illness, due to neuromuscular effects of an exotoxin *tetanospasmin,* produced by *C. tetani., a* gram-positive *anaerobe,* present as spores in stools of various herbivores animals and fecal-contaminated soil. Spores enter the body through contaminated wounds, unsterilized needles, animal bites etc. and germinate to produce a toxin - *tetanospasmin.* Toxin binds to the neuromuscular junction and traverses along the axonal sheaths towards the spinal cord to block the release of neurotransmitters in inhibitory spinal inter neurons, leading to typical muscular spasms.

Vaccines: Currently available DPT and allied vaccines may be divided into three types –

a) Vaccines used for immunization in children below 7 years e.g. DTwP, DTaP and DT;

b) Vaccines used for immunization of older children, adolescents and adults e.g. Td and TdaP

c) Monovalent Tetanus vaccine e.g. TT, used in selected conditions.

In this article, DTwP will be discussed as the prototype vaccine, followed by discussion on alternative vaccines of same class.

10.1: WHOLE-CELL PERTUSSIS DPT (DTwP)

It is available as a stand-alone triple antigen vaccine or in combination with other antigens as Quadrivalent (with HiB, HBV or IPV), Pentavalent (with HBV+HiB) or Hexavalent (with HiB, HBV and IPV) combination vaccines. Some countries have replaced DTwP with acellular DTaP due to concerns of side effects.

Contents & Storage: Each dose of DTwP contains Diphtheria toxoid ~25 Lf (flocculation limits) Tetanus toxoid ~5 Lf and killed whole-cell pertussis bacilli (20,000 million or ~4 IU). It is available as single dose ampoule (0.5 ml) or multi-dose vials and should be stored at 2–8°C.

Dosage & administration: DTwP is given as 0.5 ml/dose intramuscularly over antero-lateral side of mid-thigh or in deltoid region in older children.

Immunization Schedule: In NIS, DTwP is given as a component of Pentavalent vaccine (DTwP+HBV+HiB) for primary immunization at *6, 10 and 14 week of life*, followed by two boosters of stand-alone DTwP at *16-24 months* and *5-6 years*. Under NIS, Pentavalent vaccine is given only up to 1 year, though second/third dose may be given after 1 year only, if the first dose was given before 1 year.

IAP also recommends three primary doses of DTwP either alone or in combination at 6, 10, and 14 weeks of life with two boosters at 15–18 months and 4–5 years. Last primary dose should be given before 6 months of age and the first booster may be administered as early as at 12 months of age, provided at least 6 months have lapsed since the third dose.

Catch-up immunization below 7 years includes three doses of stand-alone DTwP at 0, 1 and 6 months with a booster dose after 6 months of the last primary dose. Second booster is not required, if the last dose has been given beyond the age of 4 years.

DTwP vaccine should not be used beyond 7 years of age for boosters or catch-up immunization due to increased risk of side effects. Low diphtheria TdaP/Td should be used in these cases, discussed later.

Efficacy: Antibody titers of > 0.1 IU/ml and > 0.01 IU/ml are considered as immunological correlates of Protection for Diphtheria and Tetanus respectively and Immunogenicity as well as Protective efficacy of DTwP against these two diseases is reported to exceed 95% after three primary doses. Disease may occur in vaccinated individuals, but in milder forms.

Protection against *B. pertussis* involves both humoral and cellular responses and no absolute or surrogate immunological correlates of protection are known for Pertussis vaccines. *Murine intracerebral challenge test* has been considered as a 'gold standard' to assess the potency of wP vaccines. Protective efficacy of DTwP against pertussis is highly variable, ranging from 46% to 98% with a pooled efficacy of 78%.

Immunity against all three components wanes over the next 6–12 years unless boosted periodically and may lead to shift in the epidemiology of disease towards older age groups.

Safety: Side-effects are mainly due to pertussis fraction and include:

a. *Local reactions* with pain and swelling in over 50% cases, usually for 24-36 hours and may be relieved with cold compresses.

b. *Transient fever* during first 24 hours in about 50% cases, which may be prevented or treated with a simple antipyretic, e.g. paracetamol. High fever > 40.5°C has been reported in 0.2–4.4/1000 vaccine doses, which may precipitate febrile seizures.

c. *Rare but serious neurological events* include persistent or inconsolable cry or screaming episodes (4.0-8.8/1000 doses), Hypotonic-hyporesponsive episodes (0.06-0.08/1000 doses), seizures (0.16-0.39/1000 doses) and encephalopathy (0.007/1000 doses).

Frequency of systemic reactions reduces and that of local reactions increases with increasing order of doses.

Adverse events e.g. sudden infant death syndrome, Infantile spasms, Autism, Learning disorders, chronic neurological damage and Reye syndrome, once attributed to DTwP are no longer considered as causally related. There have been isolated case reports of brachial neuritis after DTwP vaccine, perhaps due to faulty technique.

Persistent cry *or screaming episodes,* is defined as more than one hour of continuous, inconsolable cry within 24 hours of vaccination. Although known to occur even after DT vaccination, persistent cry is ~4 times more common following DTwP and more frequently after the first dose. Recurrence is unlikely after susbsequent doses.

Seizures following DTwP vaccination are generally febrile seizures, occurring within 3 days of vaccination. These seizures are generally benign, more common in children with a past history or family history of seizures and do not result in epilepsy.

Dravet's syndrome (Severe myoclonic epilepsy of infancy) is an epileptic encephalopathy with underlying genetic etiology (sodium channel $\alpha 1$ subunit gene or SCN1A abnormalities), which often presents with post-vaccination seizures as first manifestation in 58% cases. Seizures following vaccinations have been reported in 27% of cases with Dravet's syndrome.

Hypotonic–hyporesponsive episodes are defined as the sudden onset of limpness, reduced responsiveness and pallor or cyanosis within 48 hours of immunization. While most cases occur after pertussis containing vaccines, including acellular ones, rare cases have been reported with others e.g. pneumococcal vaccines. Exact cause is not known but recovery occurs spontaneously and no long term sequelae have been documented. Majority of these infants can be safely given further doses without recurrence.

Encephalopathy. Association of DTwP and acute serious acute neurological illness within 7 days of vaccination has been an issue of intense scrutiny, though a causal relationship cannot be ruled out. National Childhood Encephalopathy Study from UK (1976-79) reported acute encephalopathy at a rate of 1 per 310,000 to 5,300,000 DTwP doses, though subsequent studies did not demonstrate increased mortality or neurological sequelae after DTwP vaccination. In 1994, the Institute of medicine concluded that *"the balance of evidence is consistent with a causal relationship between DTwP and chronic nervous system dysfunction in children whose serious acute neurological illness occurred within 7 days of a DTwP vaccination"*. It has been suggested that the vaccine may trigger a neurological event in the individuals predisposed to develop it due to some underlying abnormality. Recent studies have concluded that DTwP vaccination is not associated with increased risk of encephalopathy.

Contraindications: *History of anaphylaxis or Encephalopathy within 7 days of previous dose is the only absolute contraindication for further dose,* due to uncertainty of the causative component. In cases of encephalopathy following vaccination, any pertussis containing vaccine is contraindicated and only diphtheria and tetanus vaccines (DT/Td) may be used for further doses, if needed.

Presence of progressive neurological illness is a *relative contraindication* to the first dose of DTwP, though it can be safely given to children with stable neurologic disorders.

Persistent inconsolable cry for >3 hrs,, Hyperpyrexia >40.5°C, Hypotonic–hyporesponsive episodes within 48 hours, and seizures with/without fever within 72 hours, are considered as *precautions but not the contraindications* to future doses of DTwP. It is advisable to observe these children for longer period after vaccination.

10.2: ACELLULAR PERTUSSIS DPT (DTaP)

DTaP vaccines have been developed to minimize the side-effects of DTwP by removal of the bacterial cell wall during the purification process and using selected bacterial antigens for the immunological challenge. All DTaP vaccines differ from one-another in terms of the number of antigens, bacterial strains used to extract them, processing techniques and use of adjuvants or preservatives and hence, should not be considered as a single product.

Contents & Storage: DTaP vaccines contain one or more of the following five separately purified pertussis antigens— pertussis toxin (PT), filamentous hemagglutinin (FHA), pertactin (PRN), and fimbrial hemagglutinins 2 and 3 (FIM type 2 and 3), apart from Diphtheria and Tetanus toxoids. These vaccines are usually available in combination with IPV and/or HBV+Hib vaccines. While there is no consensus about ideal antigenic composition of an acellular vaccine. none of them must contain less than two antigens (PT, FHA).

DTaP vaccines are available as stand-alone DTaP or in combination with other vaccines e.g. DTaP with IPV (Tetraxim®) with HIB+IPV (Pentaxim®), DTaP with HBV+HIB+IPV (Hexaxim®, Infanrix Hexa®)), all supplied as single-dose preparation. All DTaP vaccines must be stored at 2–8°C.

Dosage & administration: DTaP is given as 0.5 ml/dose of stand-alone or combination vaccine, Intramuscularly over antero-lateral aspect of mid-thigh.

Immunization Schedule: DTaP vaccines are not used in NIS. IAP recommends DTaP may be considered for booster doses as well as for primary series, irrespective of the number of components in view of the parental concerns regarding side-effects of DTwP. However, it recognizes that wP vaccine is definitely superior to aP vaccine in terms of immunogenicity and duration of protection.

DTaP may be specially considered for - a) Booster doses in view of the higher reactogenicity of DTwP in older children; and b) subsequent doses in cases with history of severe adverse effects after previous DTwP dose; or c) children with neurologic disorders. Like DTwP vaccines, DTaP vaccines must also not be used in children beyond 7 years of age.

Efficacy: *Protective efficacy* of DTaP vaccines against Diphtheria and Tetanus is comparable to that of DTwP i.e. over 95% after three primary doses.

Immunogenicity of DTaP against pertussis is not well established as there are no animal model to assess and unlike DTwP, these vaccines do not pass the 'murine intracerebral challenge test'. Antibody titers against PT, PRN and FIM antigens have been used as correlates of protection with inconclusive results.

In recent years, large outbreaks of pertussis have been reported in countries which shifted from DTwP to DTaP in their NIS. Similar outbreaks have been also reported in countries using DTwP, albeit rarely. These outbreaks have been linked to the declining immunity with age. Studies suggest that protective efficacy of both acellular and whole cell vaccines is comparable in the first year of vaccination but immunity wanes faster with the aP vaccines. However, the duration of protection with both vaccines is comparable after three primary doses and a booster dose at least after a year. It has been suggested that priming with DTwP is more effective than DTaP vaccines, for sustained prevention of disease.

Further, all DTaP vaccines are not same and each brand is unique in itself due to differences in the number, source and quantity of constituent antigens as well as manufacturing processes. DTaP vaccines containing three or more antigens have shown a higher efficacy (80-85%) than those containing two or less antigens (60-75%)[8], though current evidence is not enough to establish superiority of any DTaP vaccine over others based on the number of antigens. IAP recommends that all licensed DTaP vaccines are of similar efficacy and safety and anyone of them may be used.

Safety: DTaP vaccines have significant lower incidence of local pain and fever following vaccination, reduced by about two-third due to DTwP vaccines. All licensed DTaP vaccines are comparable in terms of side effects. Rate and severity of local reactions tend to increase with successive DTaP doses. Serious adverse events are also less likely with DTaP vaccines, but may occur.

Contraindications: Despite the lower risk, absolute contra-indications for DTaP vaccines are same as those for whole cell vaccines i.e. history of anaphylaxis or encephalopathy following previous dose.

10.3: BIVALENT DIPHTHERIA & TETANUS TOXOID (DT)

DT is a bivalent vaccine containing Diphtheria toxoid and Tetanus toxoid in same quantity as in DTwP/DTaP, but with-out pertussis component. This vaccine is rarely used at present except *in children below 7 years with contraindications for pertussis containing vaccines* e.g. anaphylaxis or encephalopathy with the previous dose.

10.4: TETANUS TOXOID WITH LOW-DOSE DIPHTHERIA TOXOID VACCINE (Td)

Till recently, TT was widely used for wound management and decennial booster dose to protect against potential exposures, as antibody titers are known to decline over time. Diphtheria antibody titers are also known to decline similarly, though adequate childhood coverage (> 70%) was expected to provide herd effect to prevent outbreaks in adults. However, recent surveillance data has shown that majority of diphtheria cases in India are currently reported in older children beyond five years of age (77% in 2017, 69% in 2018), underscoring the need for diphtheria boosters, along with Tetanus booster.

Since 1998, WHO has recommended that TT should be replaced by Td vaccine and India has gradually introduced it in NIS since 2018.

Content & Storage: Td is a bivalent vaccine containing lower dose of diphtheria toxoid (2-5 Lf instead of 25 Lf) along with the usual dose of Tetanus toxoid (> 5 Lf) without pertussis component. It should be stored at 2–8°C.

Dosage & administration: Td vaccine is given intramuscularly as 0.5 ml/ dose over deltoid region.

Immunization schedule: In NIS, Td has replaced TT since 2018, as follows -

a) *Pregnant women:* Two doses (Td_1 & Td_2) 4 weeks apart starting in early pregnancy. Single dose booster (Td_b) is needed during subsequent pregnancy, if two doses were received in last pregnancy within past 3 years.

b) *Children:* Two booster doses at 10 and 16 years.

IAP also recommends Td to replace TT in all situations including -

a) Catch-up immunization beyond 7 years of age, preferably after the first dose of Tdap (discussed later, also see FAQ 7);

b) Booster doses every 10 years in fully immunized children.

c) Wound care

Safety: Side-effects are rare except local pain, though boosters may lead to increased frequency and severity of local and systemic reactions as the preformed antitoxin binds with the toxoid and leads to immune complex-mediated reactions (swollen limbs and Arthus type-2 reactions).

Contraindications are none.

10.5: TETANUS TOXOID WITH LOW-DOSE DIPHTHERIA TOXOID & ACELLULAR PERTUSSIS VACCINE (TDaP)

Immunity against pertussis following DTwP/DTaP vaccination wanes over the next 6–12 years and recent years have seen substantial rise in pertussis among older children, adolescents and adults due to expanding immunization coverage in early childhood and consequent shift in the age-epidemiology. Pertussis in older age is not only associated with higher morbidity but also serves as a reservoir for transmission to unvaccinated infants.

However, regular DTwP and DTaP vaccines cannot be used for vaccination of children 7 years and above due to increased reactogenicity of high antigenic contents of Diphtheria and pertussis antigens in them. TdaP is the triple vaccine recommended for immunization of older children, adolescents and adults. Lower case letters "d" and "p" in the nomenclature of this vaccine indicates lower concentration of diphtheria and pertussis toxoids, while "a" indicates acellular pertussis component.

Contents & Storage: Tdap contains lower dose of diphtheria toxoid (2.5 Lf instead of 25 Lf) as well as less than half of the doses of pertussis antigens as compared to DTaP, along with usual strength of Tetanus toxoid.

Tdap vaccines (Boosterix®, Adacel®) are available as single dose liquid 0.5 ml, usually in prefilled syringes, which should be stored at 2–8°C.

Dosage & administration: Tdap vaccine is to be given intramuscularly (0.5 ml) over deltoid region.

Immunization schedule: Although not included in the NIS, IAP recommends a single one-time dose of Tdap instead of Td/TT vaccines to -

a) All adolescents at 11-12 years, if fully immunized previously,

b) All pregnant women preferably during 27-36 weeks, irrespectively of Td/TdaP doses in previous pregnancy.

c) Unimmunized persons above 7 years, as the first dose for catch-up immunization followed by two further doses of Td at one month and six month interval (0, 1, 6 month). Catch-up vaccination is recommended till the age of 18 years.

d) Partially immunized persons above 7 years, as the first catch-up dose, followed by Td as remaining doses, if needed.

Adolescent dose should not be given, if the catch-up Tdap dose was used. In fact, *more than one dose of TdaP is not recommended, except in pregnancy.*

Efficacy: Immunogenicity studies have shown that antibody response to a single dose of Tdap booster in previously vaccinated person is similar to that following three primary doses of DTwP or DTaP. Protective efficacy against clinical disease is about 66-78%, though may exceed 90%. Effectiveness wanes within 3–4 years and there is no evidence of herd immunity.

Safety: Commonest side-effect is the local pain at injection site in ~70% vaccinees, followed by redness and swelling. Systemic side effects like fever, headache and fatigue are rare. Serious adverse events have not been reported.

Contraindications include serious allergic reaction or encephalopathy within seven days of administration of any vaccine with pertussis component, not attributable to an underlying cause.

10.6: MONOVALENT TETANUS TOXOID VACCINE (TT)

TT, used till recently for booster doses at 10 and 16 years and during pregnancy, has been gradually replaced with Td/Tdap vaccine, discussed earlier. Currently, it is mainly used for wound management.

Content & Storage: TT is a monovalent vaccine, containing Tetanus toxoid (5 Lf), adsorbed on aluminium phosphate. It is available as a single dose (0.5 ml) or in multi-dose vials, to be stored at 2–8°C. It is one of the most heat stable vaccine.

Dosage & administration: TT is given intramuscularly (0.5 ml) over deltoid region or on anterolateral aspect of thigh in young children.

Immunization schedule: TT is no longer used in NIS, replaced with Td for pregnant mothers and boosters beyond 10 years. Moreover, it is also recommended that the TT doses given during wound management should also be replaced with

Td or other age-appropriate tetanus containing vaccines as per previous immunization status, for more comprehensive protection.

Side effects are rare except transient local pain and local reactions in ~50% vaccinees. Systemic reactions e.g. fever, malaise and shivering may occur in 1-2% cases, specially in older age groups. Administration of boosters more frequently than indicated, leads to increased frequency and severity of local and systemic reactions as the preformed antitoxin binds with the toxoid and leads to immune complex-mediated reactions (swollen limbs and Arthus type 2 reactions).

Contraindications are none, except allergy to previous dose of Tetanus containing vaccine.

Frequently Asked Questions (FAQs)

1. **Which vaccine is preferable for early childhood immunization – DTwP or DTaP?**

    Protective efficacy of both acellular and whole cell vaccines is comparable in the first year of vaccination but the immunity wanes faster with the DTaP than DTwP; However, minor side effects e.g. local pain and fever are distinctly less common with DTaP than with DTwP. Serious adverse effects are rare even with DTwP vaccines and can still occur (albeit less commonly) with DTaP.

    Considering more sustained protection, DTwP is preferred over DtaP despite higher incidence of minor side effects, which can be easily managed. However, IAP recommends DTaP may be used for primary as well as booster doses in view of parental concerns about side-effects as long as it helps to improve immunization coverage. Though, It also recognizes that DTwP is definitely superior to DTaP in terms of immunogenicity and duration of protection.

2. **What should be the subsequent immunization practice, if a child develops anaphylaxis or encephalopathy after a DTwP dose.**

This child should be given DT (not DTaP) instead of DPT for the remaining doses, as it is usually the Pertussis component, which is responsible for serious adverse events and severe reactions may develop even after DTaP.

3. **What should be subsequent immunization, if a child develops febrile convulsions, screaming episodes or hypotonic-hyporesponsive episodes after first dose of DTwP.**

This case should continue to receive DTwP for subsequent doses, with longer period of observation. DTaP may be considered in these cases for booster doses, if resources permit.

4. **Whether a child with cerebral palsy can be given DTwP.**

Yes, since it is not a progressive neurological disease.

5. **Whether an unimmunized child recovering from confirmed Tetanus, Diphtheria or Pertussis disease, still needs DPT immunization?**

Yes. Since natural disease does not offer complete protection and the child has also to be protected against other vaccine-constituent diseases. He should be immunized after 3-4 weeks of recovery.

6. **A two year old child is unimmunized for DPT. What should be the catch-up immunization schedule for him?**

Catch-up immunization below 7 years of age involves three doses of DTwP/DTaP at 0, 1 and 6 months with a booster dose after 6 months of the last primary dose. Second booster is not required if the last dose has been given beyond 4 years age.

Under NIS, first dose of Pentavalent vaccine is given only up to 1 year, but second/third dose may be given even after that if the first dose was given before 1 year.

7. **An eight year old child is unimmunized for DPT. What should be the catch-up immunization schedule for him?**

Catch-up immunization above 7 years is recommended upto 18 years of age and includes first dose of Tdap followed by two doses of Td after one and six month (0,1,6 month).

8. **What do small case letters 'd', 'a' and 'p' represent in nomenclature of DPT vaccines?**

Small case letters "d" and "p" in the nomenclature of this vaccine indicates lower concentration of diphtheria toxoid and pertussis antigens as used in vaccines for children above 7 years (TdaP/Td), while "a" indicates acellular pertussis component.

9. **Whether DTwP and DTaP vaccines can be inter-changed?**

In principle, the same type and same brand of the vaccine should be given throughout the whole schedule, though brands can be interchanged, if unavoidable. IAP also permits change from DTwP primary schedule to DTaP for boosters, if resources permit. Change from DTaP to DTwP is usually requested due to unaffordability and may be permitted. Change from DTwP to DTaP is usually requested due to side effects and parents must be counseled about benefits of DTwP and possibility of similar side effects with DtaP, though less common. Switch from DTwP to DTaP should not be encouraged for primary doses.

10. **Whether a fully immunized child till second booster also needs Tdap.**

A single one-time dose of Tdap is recommended to all fully immunized children at 11-12 years (instead of

10 year TT/TD booster) as Immunity against pertussis, even after boosters, wanes over the next 6–12 years and recent years have seen substantial rise in cases of pertussis among older children, adolescents and adults. Pertussis in these older age groups is not only associated with higher morbidity but also serves as a reservoir for disease transmission to unvaccinated infants.

11. **What is the role of Tetanus toxoid and Tetanus immunoglobulins in wound management?**

Tetanus spores, usually present in fecal-contaminated soil, enter the body largely via contaminated wounds and prevention of tetanus in such cases involves- a) local wound care, b) Tetanus immunoglobulins and c) Tetanus containing vaccines.

Local wound care involves cleaning, irrigation, drainage and removal of devitalized tissue, as required, to prevent anaerobic environment conducive of toxin production.

Passive prophylaxis with Tetanus Immunoglobulin (TIG 250 -500 IU IM) is necessary, irrespective of the wound severity, only in cases with - a) unknown immunization status, b) Incomplete immunization with less than 3 doses of tetanus containing vaccines, and c) Immunodeficiency states.

Tetanus toxoid containing vaccines (DTwP/Tdap/Td) with choice depending on the age, feasibility and previous doses received, if any, are recommended as follows –

- Fully immunized persons with at least three doses must receive a single booster dose, if the last dose was received 5 years back (10 years for clean/minor wounds);

- Partially immunized children should be given the next due dose, followed by subsequent dose (if required) to complete at least three doses counting previous dose/s.

- Unimmunized persons (or those with unknown immunization history) should receive three doses depending on the age at 0,1,6 months to complete the immunization

12. What is the need for Tdap/Td immunization in pregnant mothers?

Antibody titers against Tetanus and Diphtheria after childhood immunization wane over time and may drop below protective levels. While TT was widely used for antenatal immunization to cover perinatal risks, it has been replaced with Td in the NIS since 2018, to use this opportunity for simultaneous booster of diphtheria immunity in fully immunized women and provide/complete necessary doses in unimmunized or partially immunized women.

Although not included in the NIS, IAP recommends a single dose of Tdap instead of Td in all pregnancies to ensure adequate transplacental antibody transfer to protect the newborn till his/her own immunization.

13. What are the recommendations for antenatal immunization?

WHO recommends that all previously unimmunized pregnant women should receive two doses – first dose of Tdap/Td at the time of first-contact and the second dose of Td after one month and at least 2 weeks before the delivery. A single dose of Tdap/Td should be administered in each subsequent pregnancy. However, fully immunized mothers with all primary doses and boosters, including Adolescent Tdap, need only one dose in each pregnancy.

NIS has replaced TT with Td since 2018, with two doses (Td1 and Td2) at four weeks interval starting in early pregnancy. Single dose booster (Td_b) is needed during subsequent pregnancy within 3 years of last pregnancy, provided, two Td doses were received in last pregnancy.

Key Points

Vaccine: D & T toxoids + Whole cell/acellular Pertussis in different combinations

Dose: 0.5 ml/dose for all combinations

Immunization Schedule:

Childhood Immunization:

NIS: DTwP - 3 doses at 6,10,14 weeks, Booster at 16-24 mo and 5-6 yrs, Td at 10,16 years (given as Pentavalent vaccine with HBV and HIB)

IAP: DTwP/DTaP - 3 doses at 6,10,14 weeks, Booster at 15-18 mo and 4-5 yrs, Tdap 11-12 yr (preferably as Pentavalent/ hexavalent vaccine)

Catch-up Immunization:

< 7 yrs: DTwP at 0, 1, 6 mo, Booster after 6 mo. (No Booster if last dose given > 4 yrs age)

> 7 yrs: Tdap/Td followed by 2 doses of Td at 0, 1, 6 mo (No Tdap booster at 11-12 years).

Pregnancy:

NIS: Td at 0, 1 mo. last dose at least 2 wk before first delivery (single dose in next Pregnancies)

IAP: Tdap single dose in all pregnancies (with Td as second dose after 1 mo in first pregnancy)

Efficacy: Diphtheria & Tetanus >95%, Pertussis 70-80%

Safety: Local reactions and Fever (more with whole-cell pertussis vaccines) *Rare:* persistent cry, HHE, Seizures, Encephalopathy

Contraindications: H/o anaphylaxis, encephalopathy with previous dose

---

IAP recommends that all pregnant women should receive a one-time dose of Tdap instead of Td, preferably during 27-36 weeks, irrespectively of previous Td/TdaP dose and this dose is necessary in every pregnancy

14. A fully-immunized girl including Tdap at 16 years, gets pregnant at 19 years. Whether she need Tdap/Td during pregnancy?

All fully immunized pregnant women, even including adolescent Tdap/Td, should receive a single dose of Tdap/Td in each pregnancy.

15. Whether it is safe and appropriate to give Tdap in pregnancy?

Although the safety data with Tdap administration during pregnancy is limited at present, even multiple doses of wP vaccines during pregnancy have not observed serious untoward events. There is a concern that maternal pertussis immunization may interfere with uptake of pertussis vaccines during primary immunization due to higher concentrations of transplacentally transferred maternal antibodies. However, studies have shown that despite some blunting of the initial response to the infant series, children develop adequate antibodies by the end of the complete series

References

1. World Health Organization, Diphtheria vaccines. Position paper, Wkly Epidemiol Rec. 2017;92:417-436
2. World Health Organization, Tetanus vaccines. Position paper, Wkly Epidemiol Rec. 2017;92: 53-76
3. World Health Organization. Pertussis vaccines: Position paper. Wkly Epidemiol Rec. 2015;90:433-60.
4. Pallab Chatterjee. Diphtheria, Tetanus and Pertussis vaccines *In:* IAP Guidebook on Immunization 2018-19 - Advisory Committee on Vaccines and Immunization Practices, Indian Academy of Pediatrics, 3rd Edition, New Delhi, Jaypee Brothers 2020; pp 134-159.
5. Choudhary SK et al. Diphtheria, Tetanus and Pertussis *In:* Vashishtha V et al. FAQs on Vaccines and immunization practices. 2nd Edition. New Delhi, Jaypee Brothers 2015; pp 127-144.
6. Introduction of Td vaccine in Universal Immunization Programme of India - Operational Guidelines: Available from: https://nhm.gov.in/New_Updates_2018/NHM_Components/Immunization/Guildelines_for_immunization/Td_vaccine_operational_guidelines.pdf (accessed on 20th June, 2021)
7. Ministry of Health and Family welfare, Government of India. National Immunization Schedule and Frequently asked questions *In:* Immunization Handbook for health workers 2018; pp 17-26.
8. Jefferson et al. Systemic review of the effects of pertussis vaccines in children. Vaccine. 2003;21:2003-14.

11 | H. Influenzae B Vaccine

H. influenzae b (Hib) infection is the commonest cause of meningitis and pneumonia in young children of developing countries, though the disease has nearly disappeared from western world due to widespread immunization. Exact burden of Hib disease in India is not well established though estimated to be severe enough to warrant routine immunization.

Epidemiology: *H. influenzae,* is a gram-negative coccobacilli in capsulated or uncapsulated forms, with six serotypes (a–f). Invasive disease e.g. pneumonia and meningitis, is almost always caused by *capsulated serotype b*, while other serotypes and uncapsulated organisms may cause localized airway disease e.g. bronchitis, otitis, sinusitis etc. or the invasive disease in immunocompromized host. Uncapsulated Hib disease is not preventable at present and can occur at any age.

Hib colonize respiratory flora via droplet infections with colonization rate being directly related to age. Uncolonized young infants are most susceptible for Hib disease and >90% cases of invasive disease occur within first 5 years of life. Disease is very rare beyond this age, except in immunocompromized children, specially those with *splenic dysfunction,* e.g. sickle cell disease, asplenia and splenectomy.

Vaccines: Hib Vaccine (HIB) is available as a stand-alone vaccine as well in combination with DTwP/DTaP with or without HBV and/or IPV. In NIS, HIB vaccine is given as a part of pentavalent vaccine, along with DPT and HBV.

All HIB vaccines are conjugated vaccines, containing a purified capsular polysaccharide (polyribosylribitol phosphate or PRP), conjugated with a carrier protein to boost the immunogenicity. Depending on the carrier protein, three types of vaccines are available—HbOC (carrier mutant *C. diphtheria* toxin), PRP-T (carrier tetanus toxoid) and PRP-OMP (carrier *N. meningitidis* outer membrane protein complex). PRP-OMP is not available in India at present.

Contents & storage: Stand-alone HIB vaccines are single dose (10 µg/0.5 ml) lyophilized vaccines, supplied with diluents and need to be reconstituted before use. Combination vaccines containing Hib are liquid vaccines, which do not require reconstitution. All vaccines need to be stored at 2–8°C.

Dosage & Administration: HIB vaccine is given intramuscularly as 0.5 ml/dose over antero-lateral thigh in infants or deltoid region in older children, if not given earlier.

Immunization Schedule: Minimum age to start HIB vaccine is 6 weeks. In NIS, Hib vaccine is given as Pentavalent vaccine (DPT+HBV+HIB) with three doses at 6, 10 and 14 weeks of age, *without any booster dose.*

IAP also recommends three primary doses as in NIS but also *followed by one booster dose at 12–18 months.*

Catch-up immunization depends on the age of vaccinee at the time of first visit, as follows -

- *6–12 months:* Two primary doses at 0, 1 month followed by one booster dose at 12-18 months, at least 8 weeks after second dose.

- *12–15 months:* One primary dose followed by one booster dose after at least 8 weeks.

- 15 months - 5 years : Single dose, no booster

No catch-up immunization is recommended beyond 5 years of age due to rarity of HiB infection, except in *high-risk children or adults* e.g. those with asplenia, hyposplenia splenectomy etc, who should receive a single dose of HIB vaccine, if not immunized earlier. Recipients of stem cell transplant should be revaccinated according to their age, regardless of previous Hib vaccination history.

Efficacy: Serologic titers of 0.15 µg/ml and 1 µg/ml are considered as correlates of protection for Hib infection at the time of exposure and for long-term protection, respectively. Antibody titers rise marginally after the first dose but rapidly reach the protective threshold after subsequent doses.

Studies have shown a protective efficacy of 90–100% for at least one year against culture-proven invasive HiB disease. However, Immunity wanes over time and reduced carriage of the organism in the population after widespread immunization prevents natural boosting. As the immunological memory following primary doses may be insufficient for long-term protection, IAP recommends a booster dose at 12-18 months, though it is not included in NIS.

HIB Vaccine also provides herd protection by reducing the nasopharyngeal carriage of organism, even to unimmunized children.

Safety: Side-effects are rare except transient mild fever and local reactions in 5-30% cases.

Contraindications: None, though the dose may be deferred during acute severe febrile illness.

Frequently Asked Questions (FAQs)

1. **Which HIB Vaccine is more effective and safe?**

   Both available HIB vaccines in India (HbOC and PRP-T) are equally effective and safe. While PRP-OMP vaccine is more rapidly immunogenic and needs only two primary doses, it is not presently available in India.

2. **Why HIB immunization is not recommended after 5 years of age?**

   Over >90% cases of invasive Hib disease occur within first 5 years of life. Disease is very rare beyond this age, except in high-risk children.

3. **Why a booster is recommended by IAP, when it is not a part of national immunization schedule?**

   Vaccine-induced Immunity wanes over time and reduced carriage of the organism in the population after universal immunization prevents natural boosting. Some countries reported surge of Hib disease among vaccinated children after initial decline, usually at the end of second year. As the immunological memory following primary doses may be insufficient for long-term protection, IAP recommends a booster dose at 12-18 months, though it is not included in UIP.

4. **Who needs HIB immunization beyond 5 years of age?**

   Older children and adults with *splenic dysfunction*, e.g. Asplenia, functional hyposplenism (e.g. sickle cell disease) or those undergoing splenectomy are at risk of Hib infection and need immunization, if not immunized earlier. Recipients of stem cell transplant should also be re-vaccinated, regardless of previous HIB vaccination.

5. **How many doses are required for high-risk older population?**

   Only one dose is required *without booster* in high-risk population above 5 years of age.

6. **When should a 10-year old child undergoing planned splenectomy be vaccinated with HiB vaccine? Can he receive it with other pre-splenectomy vaccines?**

Any person undergoing elective splenectomy must receive single dose of HIB vaccine at least 2 weeks prior to surgery, which can be given along with other vaccines.

7. **An adolescent, unimmunized for Hib earlier, needed emergency splenectomy due to an automobile accident. When should he be immunized with Hib vaccine?**

He should be immunized preferably after 2 weeks of surgery for appropriate immune response.

8. **Whether this vaccine can be used for Post-exposure prophylaxis in close contacts?**

No. Post exposure prophylaxis is indicated only in un-immunized children < 5 years of age or high-risk factors following close contact with a documented Hib Case, with PO *Rifampicin* (10–20 mg/kg OD for 4 days). It is also necessary to eliminate carrier state in index Case.

Key Points

- **Vaccine:** Conjugated, stand-alone or Combination Vaccine
- **Dose:** IM 0.5 ml/dose (1ml >18 yrs age, if required)
- **Schedule:**
  - *NIS:* Total 3 primary doses at 6, 10 & 14 weeks, No boosters
  - *IAP:* Total 3 primary doses at 6, 10 & 14 weeks with Booster at 12–18 months
- **Catch-up immunization:** Upto 5 years (upto 1 year in NIS)
  - 6–12 mo: Two primary doses at 0, 1 mo, Booster at 12–18 mo (8 weeks after last primary dose)
  - 12–15 mo: Single primary dose, Booster after 8 weeks
  - Above 15 mo: Single dose, No booster
  - High-risk cases not immunized earlier: Single dose, no booster.
- **Protective efficacy:** >90% for 1–2 years against culture proven invasive disease, Herd effect.
- **Side effects** rare, except Local reaction or mild fever
- **Contraindications:** None, may be deferred in acute severe febrile illness.

References

1. World Health Organization. Hemophilus influenza type B vaccines. Position paper. Weekly Epid. Record 2013;88: 413-428.
2. Shivananda S. Haemophilus Influenzae Type B conjugate vaccine *In:* IAP Guidebook on Immunization 2018-19 - Advisory Committee on Vaccines and Immunization Practices, Indian Academy of Pediatrics, 3rd Edition, New Delhi, Jaypee Brothers 2020; pp 160-167.
3. Choudhury J. Haemophilus Influenzae Type B vaccine *In:* Vashishtha V et al. FAQs on Vaccines and immunization practices. 2nd Edition. New Delhi, Jaypee Brothers 2015; pp 215-219.
4. Ministry of Health and Family welfare, Government of India. National Immunization Schedule and Frequently asked questions *In*: Immunization Handbook for health workers 2018; pp 17-26.

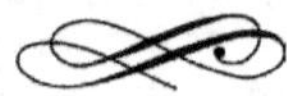

Rotavirus Vaccines

Rotavirus associated gastroenteritis (RVGE) is leading cause of severe diarrhea in infants and toddlers, accounting for ~5% of global deaths in under-five children. In India, RVGE accounts for 35-40% of diarrhea-related hospitalizations with stool positivity rate of 20-40% in hospitalized children.

Rotavirus (RV) immunization was not favored till the turn of this century due to potential risk of intussusceptions observed with an earlier licensed vaccine 'Rotashield' in 1998-99. However, with availability of safer vaccines now, RV vaccine has been gradually introduced in NIS since 2016.

Epidemiology: RV is an RNA virus with seven serogroups (A–G). Most human cases are due to group A virus. Outer viral capsid is made up of VP7 and VP4 proteins, which determines G and P serotypes respectively. While all G serotypes correspond with G genotypes, P serotypes have more genotypes than serotypes. Each strain is designated by its G serotype followed by P serotype and then P genotype number in square brackets. In India, most common RV strains are G1P[8] accounting for 62.7% cases, followed by G2P[4], G1P[4], G12P[6] and G9P[8], last two being more common in recent years.

Protective immunity against RV involves both humoral and cellular components. After first infection, serological response is directed mainly against the specific viral serotype (*homotypic response*), while subsequent infections lead to broader, *heterotypic antibody response* reducing, albeit not necessarily, the risk and severity of further infections.

Majority of RVGE cases occur in first two years of life, though re-infections or even the first episode may be delayed until the age of 2–5 years. Infection is transmitted via feco-oral route, direct person to person contact or fomites and probably by other routes e.g. droplets.Unlike seasonal (winter) trend in temperate countries, Infection is perennial in India and re-infections are common.

Vaccines: All currently available RV vaccines are live attenuated vaccines, with four types – (a) Human monovalent vaccine (RV1), (b) Human-bovine monovalent vaccine (RHBV1), (c) Human-bovine Pentavalent vaccine (RV5), and (d) Pentavalent bovine-human reassortant vaccine (BRV-PV).

RV1 *(Rotarix®)* is derived from the human 89-12 strain of G1P[8] type, propagated on Vero cells with each reconstituted dose containing at least 10^6 median CCID50 of live attenuated virus.

RHBV1 *(Rotavac® Rotasure®)* is a live, naturally attenuated vaccine containing monovalent, bovine human reassortant strain characterized as G9 P [11] with the VP4 of bovine origin, and all other segments of human rotavirus origin. This strain was isolated from asymptomatic infants with mild diarrhea by Indian researchers in 1985 at AIIMS, New Delhi. Each dose (0.5 ml) contains not less than 10^5 FFU of live rotavirus.

RV5 *(Rotateq®)* is a Human bovine reassortant vaccine, containing five reassortants between the bovine WC23 strain and human G1, G2, G3, G4 and P1A[8] strains grown in vero cells with each 2-ml vial dose containing ~ 2×10^6 infectious units of each reassortant strains.

BRV-PV *(Rotasiil®)* is a live attenuated pentavalent bovine-human reassortant vaccine containing five single gene substitution reassortants between human strains G1, G2, G3, G4, and G9 and the bovine UK strain, grown on vero cells. Each dose contains $\geq 10^{5.6}$ FFU of each serotype. These strains were developed by the US National Institutes of Health and licensed to several emerging-country manufacturers, including India.

Contents & storage: RV1 and BRV-PV are lyophilized vaccines supplied with the diluents and need to be administered promptly after reconstitution. Diluents contain Calcium carbonate for RV1 and Citrated Sodium bicarbonate for BRV-PV.

RV5 and RHBV1 are liquid vaccines and do not need reconstitution. RV5 is suspended in a buffer solution while RHBV1 does not contain any buffer.

All vaccines must be stored at 2–8°C and not be frozen. BRV-PV vaccine is *thermo-stable* at 25°C for 30 months, 37°C for 24 months and 40°C for 6 months.

Dosage & Administration: All vaccines are given orally with variable volume/dose - 1 ml for reconstituted RV1, 2 ml for RV5, 0.5 ml for RHBV1 and 2.5 ml of reconstituted BRV-PV. Under NIS, 5 drops of RHBV1 vaccine is given per dose.

Immunization Schedule: No rotavirus vaccine should be given before 6 weeks. RV1 is a 2-dose vaccine given at one month interval, preferably at 10 and 14 weeks. All others are 3-dose vaccines, given at 6,10,14 weeks. Interchange of vaccines should be avoided or if unavoidable, total 3 doses must be given in any case (even if the first dose was RV1).

In NIS, Three doses of RHBV1 are given at 6,10,14 weeks of age.

Catch-up immunization: In NIS, upper age limit for the first dose of RV vaccine is one year. If the child has received first dose by 12 months of age, two subsequent doses should be given at monthly interval to complete the course. WHO recommends RV vaccine up to 2 years of age.

However, IAP recommends that RV vaccination should not be initiated at or after 15 weeks of age due to insufficient safety data and all doses must be completed by 32 weeks. Vaccination should be avoided, if age of the infant is uncertain.

Efficacy: All vaccines are equally immunogenic and protective despite different compositions. Protective efficacy of RV vaccines is generally measured in terms of their ability to prevent severe Rotavirus Gastroenteritis events (SRVGE)., as these vaccines are relatively less efficacious against mild infection.

Reported protective efficacy of RV1 and RV5 vaccines against SRVGE is ~80-90% in developed countries and relatively less i.e. ~50-60% in developing countries including India, perhaps due to widely prevalent malnutrition, co-infections with other enteral pathogens, interference due to high levels of maternal antibodies or presence of anti-rotavirus neutralizing antibodies in breast milk. Protective efficacy of RHBV1 and BRV-PV is also ~50-60% against SRVG. Protection generally lasts through 2nd year of life. Protective value declines if RV vaccines are given in second year of life than in infancy.

Despite the lower efficacy in RV vaccines in developing countries, public health benefits in terms of the numbers of severe disease and deaths averted by RV vaccines are much higher due to higher incidence of SRVGE.

Observational studies in developing countries have shown 30-35% reduction in all diarrhea-related deaths after introduction of RV vaccines.

Safety: Side-effects are rare except a definite but very small risk of acute intussusception (~ 1–2/lac doses), though the benefits of vaccination far exceed the miniscule risk. Risk is higher after the first dose.

Contraindications are none except past history of intussusceptions (absolute contraindication), allergy to the previous dose or Severe combined immunodeficiency. Vaccine may be given during minor illnesses but deferred during acute gastroenteritis episode due to potential compromise of uptake. Infants with latex allergy should not receive RV1 vaccine, in which a latex oral applicator is used.

Safety and efficacy of RV vaccines in infants with chronic gastrointestinal disease, gut malformations, previous intussusceptions and immunocompromised infants is not established and risk-benefit ratio must be considered.

Frequently Asked Questions (FAQs)

1. **Whether RV vaccine can be given to preterms?**

   Despite relatively uncertain efficacy and safety, RV vaccination is advised to all preterms after 6 weeks of age, if clinically stable, as they are more susceptible to severe RVGE.

2. **Till what age the catch-up immunization is recommended if missed at due date?**

   Upper age limit for the first dose of RV vaccine is 12 months under NIS (with two subsequent doses at monthly interval) and 15 weeks as per IAP schedule (with last dose before 32 weeks). However, WHO recommends RV vaccine up to 2 years of age.

3. **Why should RV vaccine be avoided in older children?**

   RV vaccine is not advised beyond the recommended upper age limits as – a) RVGE is uncommon after 2nd birthday, b) Protective value declines if vaccine is given after first year of life and c) higher risk of intususception in older children.

4. **Which RV vaccine is preferable? Whether Pentavalent vaccines are more efficacious than monovalent vaccines?**

    All vaccines, irrespective of monovalent or pentavalent, are equally effective against SRGVE (50-60%) and safe. Though pentavalent vaccines cover 47.9% of strains versus 22.1% of strains covered by monovalent vaccines, cross-protection across genotypes has been observed with use of monovalent vaccines with comparable efficacy.

5. **Whether RV brands can inter-change if the one used for earlier dose is unavailable?**

    Interchange of vaccine brand should be avoided. However, if unavoidable, then total 3 doses must be given in any case, even if the first dose was given as two-dose RV1.

6. **Whether Breast feeding should be avoided for some time after RV administration?**

    Breast feeding is not restricted before or after vaccination.

7. **Whether vaccine needs to be given again if infant regurgitates or vomits a dose?**

    Re-administration is generally not needed in such event, though some manufacturers recommend it. Remaining doses should continue as scheduled.

8. **Whether RV vaccine can be given simultaneously with OPV.**

    Yes. It can be given in same sitting either before or after OPV. Immunogenicity studies about simultaneous administration show no significant reduction for either vaccine.

9. **Whether RV vaccines are safe?**

    All RV vaccines are safe except a definite but very rare risk of acute intussusception (~1–2/lac vaccines). Risk is higher after the first dose.

10. **Will RV vaccination prevent all diarrhea?**

    It is advisable to explain to the parents that RV vaccine prevents severe diarrhea due to RV only and not due to other causes. Baby may still get diarrhea due to other causes or even mild diarrhea due to RV, especially if hygiene is overlooked.

11. **Whether vaccine can be given during acute diarrhea?**

    Yes, though efficacy of this dose may be doubtful, like any other oral vaccine dose.

12. **Whether diluents, other than that supplied with vaccine can be used in case of RV1 or BRV-PV vaccines, if required (RV5 and RHBV1 are ready-to-use liquid vaccines, which do not need reconstitution).**

    No. Diluents are vaccine specific i.e. Calcium carbonate for RV1 and Citrated Sodium bicarbonate for BRV-PV and only these should be used.

Key Points

- **Vaccine:** Live attenuated Monvalent (RV1 & RHBV1) or Pentavalent (RV5 & BRV-PV).
- **Formulation:** Lyophilized (RV1 & BRV-PV) or Liquid (RV5 & RHBV1)
- **Dose:** PO   RV1..1 ml,   RV5.. 2 ml,
             RHBV1.. 0.5 ml,   BRV.. PV 2 ml
       In NIS, only RHBV1 is used as 5 drops/dose
- **Schedule: (Minimum age 6 weeks)**
  - *NIS* (RHBV1 only) Three doses at 6,10 &14 weeks
  - *IAP:* Three doses at 6, 10, 14 weeks (for RV1, only two doses at 10, 14 weeks)
- **Catch-up immunization:**
  - *NIS:* First dose not above 1 year of age, complete with subsequent doses monthly.
  - *IAP:* First dose not at or above 15 weeks, complete before 32 weeks
- **Efficacy** >80% for SRVGE (50-60% in developing countries) for two years
- **Safety:** Side-effects rare, except definite but very small risk of intussusception (~ 1–2/lac)
- **Contraindications:** None, except history of intussusception, allergy to previous dose or SCID. It should be deferred during acute gastroenteritis.

References

1. World Health Organization. Rotavirus vaccines. Position paper: Weekly Epid. Record 2013;88: 49-64.
2. Ministry of Health and Family welfare, Government of India. Operational guidelines - Introduction of Rotavirus vaccine in Universal Immunization Program in India. December 2016.
3. Ministry of Health and Family welfare, Government of India. National Immunization Schedule and Frequently asked questions *In:* Immunization Handbook for health workers 2018; pp 17-26.
4. Kasi S et al. Rotavirus vaccines. *In:* IAP Guidebook on Immunization 2018-19 - Advisory Committee on Vaccines and Immunization Practices, Indian Academy of Pediatrics, 3rd Edition, New Delhi, Jaypee Brothers 2020; pp 207-226.
5. Shah N K. Rotavirus *In:* Vashishtha V et al. FAQs on Vaccines and immunization practices. 2nd Edition. New Delhi, Jaypee Brothers 2015; pp 268-276.

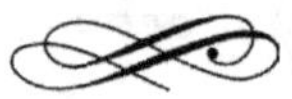

Pneumococcal Vaccines

Pneumococcal infections are common causes of morbidity and mortality in under-five children with clinical spectrum spanning from asymptomatic nasal carriage to common non-invasive illnesses e.g. sinusitis and otitis media, and serious invasive illnesses e.g. pneumonia, meningitis etc. Exact magnitude of morbidity due to pneumococcal infections is not well established in India due to difficulties in microbiological diagnosis. However, available studies suggest that pneumococci are responsible for ~12-35% of pneumonia and ~27-39% of bacterial meningitis in Indian children.

Epidemiology: *Strept. pneumoniae* is a common colonizing organism of nasopharynx with carrier rate of 27-85%, more common in under-five and institutionalized children. Infection is transmitted via droplets from a case or carrier, more common in winter season. Organism may be present in encapsulated and non-capsulated forms and only capsulated forms are pathogenic, classified according to their type-specific capsular polysaccharide. Out of over 90 serogroups, only 10 are responsible for most human infections. Invasive Pneumococcal disease (IPD) in under-five children is usually caused by serotypes 1, 5, 6, 9, 14, 19F and 23F, though the prevalence of each serotype differs with age, disease type, geographic region and changes over the time. Limited Indian data suggests that serotypes 1, 5 and 14 account for about one-third of IPD. Serotype 19A which is prevalent worldwide, causes disease in all age groups and is highly drug resistant.

Under-five children are at highest risk with about 75% cases of IPD and 83% of pneumococcal meningitis are seen in this age group, with high fatality rates. Risk factors for IPD include impaired mucociliary clearance due to preceding viral infections, passive smoking and airway allergy, malnutrition and immunodeficiency states, *specially with impaired splenic function*, e.g. sickle cell disease, asplenia, splenectomy, etc. Elderly persons above 65 years are also at risk for invasive disease,

Vaccine: Two types of pneumococcal vaccines are available - *Polysaccharide vaccine* (PPSV), used only in high-risk children and *conjugate vaccines* (PCV) recommended for universal immunization.

13.1: PNEUMOCOCCAL POLYSACCHARIDE VACCINE (PPSV)

PPSV is an unconjugated vaccine, containing capsular polysaccharide antigen from 23 serotypes (1, 2, 3, 4, 5, 6B, 7F, 8, 9N, 9V, 10A, 11A, 12F, 14,15B, 17F, 18C, 19F, 19A, 20, 22F, 23F, 33F), which are responsible for >80% cases of serious disease in adults. It is poorly immunogenic in children < 2 years and does not reduce nasopharyngeal carrier state.

Contents & storage: Vaccine is supplied as single-dose 0.5 ml suspension, containing 25 µg of each serotype antigens. It should be stored at 2-8°C.

Dosage & administration: PPSV is given as 0.5 ml/dose intramuscularly or subcutaneously over anterolateral thigh or deltoid region.

Immunization schedule: *PPSV should not be used for routine immunization of healthy children*, indicated only in high-risk children (**Table 13.1**) aged 2-18 years, along with PCV. PPSV should never be used alone for prevention of IPD in high-risk cases. All high-risk cases should receive PPSV after completing age-related PCV immunization, at least 8 weeks after the last PCV dose. Even if already vaccinated with PPSV, these cases should also receive recommended PCV doses.

Re-vaccination with PPSV is advised after 3-5 years in high-risk cases, but more than two life-time doses of PPSV is not recommended due to immunological hyporesponsiveness on repeated vaccination.

Some industrialized countries continue to use PPSV alone in the elderly and high-risk population, though WHO does not recommend it except at the discretion of the physician. IAP too does not recommend broader use of this vaccine alone in high-risk populations with underlying disease.

Efficacy: PPSV is a T-cell independent vaccine, which is poorly immunogenic below 2 years of age, has low immune memory, does not reduce nasopharyngeal carriage and does not provide herd immunity.

A single dose of PPSV23 results in the induction of sero-type-specific immunoglobulins, including IgA. Although quantitative antibody response is similar in all age groups, functional antibody response is lower in the elderly than in young adults.

Data on the protective efficacy of PPSV23 is conflicting but a systematic review has shown protective effect against IPD in healthy adults and elderly population but not in high-risk children or adults. In fact, a study from Uganda has shown higher risk of pneumonia among HIV-infected adults vaccinated with PPSV23.

Safety: Side-effects are rare except local pain and transient fever.

Contraindications include severe allergic reactions to a prior dose or to any other vaccine.

13.2: PNEUMOCOCCAL CONJUGATE VACCINE (PCV)

Currently two types of conjugate vaccines are available in India – PCV-13 containing 13 pnuemococcal antigens

(Prevenar®) or PCV-10 containing 10 antigens (synflorix® or Pneumosil®). Serotypes included in existing PCV vaccines are responsible for 49–88% of IPD related deaths in developing countries. Early generation PCV-7 is no longer available, while some PCV15 and PCV20 vaccines with higher number of serotypes are under development.

Contents & Storage: All PCV vaccines are available as single dose (0.5 ml) liquid suspension in vials/pre-filled syringes, which must be stored at 2–8°C.

PCV13 contains capsular polysaccharide antigens of 13 serotypes (1, 3, 4, 5, 6A, 6B, 7F,9V, 14, 18C, 19A, 19F, 23F), all individually conjugated to a nontoxic diphtheria cross-reactive material carrier protein (CRM197).

PCV10 contains capsular polysaccharide antigens of 10 serotypes, excluding 3 serotypes of PCV13 (3, 6A, 19A in Synflorix® and 3,4,18C in Pneumosiil®). Synflorix® uses three different carrier proteins – Tetanus toxoid, Diphtheria toxoid and non-typeable *Haemophilus influenzae* protein D for different serotypes, while in Pneumosiil® all serotypes are conjugated with nontoxic diphtheria cross-reactive material carrier protein(CRM197) as in PCV13.

Dosage & administration: All PCV vaccines are to be given as 0.5 ml/dose intramuscularly over antero-lateral thigh or deltoid region.

Immunization Schedule: In NIS, PCV has been introduced gradually since 13th May 2017, with total three doses - two primary doses as 6 and 14 weeks and a booster dose at 9 months. Upper age limit is 1 year of age. Presently, PCV10 is being used in NIS.

IAP recommends routine PCV vaccination to all infants using any PCV13/10 with total four doses – three primary doses at 6,10 and 14 weeks and a booster dose at 12–15 months of age.

Catch-up immunization is recommended till 5 years with following age-wise schedule –

- < 6 months: Three primary doses at 4 weeks interval with a booster dose at 12–15 months, at least 6 months after third dose.

- 6-12 months: Two primary doses at 4 weeks interval with a booster dose in second year.

- 12-23 months: Two primary doses at minimum 2 months interval, with No booster.

- 24-59 months: Two doses at 8 weeks interval of PCV10 or Single dose of PCV13, No booster.

PCV13 is also licensed for use as a single dose in high-risk children (6-17 years) and in adults > 50 years.

WHO recommends minimum three doses for routine childhood immunization, either as two primary doses followed by booster (2p+1) or three primary doses without boosters (3p+0). While 2p+1 schedule may leave some infants unprotected between primary and booster doses, second 3p+0 schedule may not provide long-lasting immunity beyond 18 months of age. NIS has adopted 2p+1 strategy to ensure long-term coverage.

Pneumococcal immunization of high-risk children (**Table 13.1**) is recommended only as follows –

- High-risk children aged 2-6 years with underlying medical conditions should receive single dose of PCV-13/10 (if 3 doses were received previously) *or* Two doses of PCV at least 8 weeks apart (if <3 doses were received previously), followed by single dose of PPSV at least 8 weeks after the last dose of PCV. A second dose of PPSV should be repeated after 5 years of the first dose, but more than 2 doses of PPSV are not recommended.

- High-risk children aged 6-18 years must receive single dose of PCV-13/10, followed by PPSV at least 8 weeks after the last dose of PCV. A second dose of PPSV should be repeated after 5 years of the first dose, but more than 2 doses of PPSV are not recommended.

- For planned splenectomy, cochlear implant or immuno-suppressive therapy, PCV13/10 and PPSV vaccination should be completed at least 2 weeks before surgery or initiation of therapy.

- Children who have received PPSV previously should also receive recommended PCV-13/10 doses at least 8 weeks after PPSV.

- Concurrent administration if PCV and PPSV is not recommended with minimum 8 weeks interval between two vaccines.

Table 13.1: High risk children for Pneumococcal vaccination

Immunocompetent children with
- Chronic heart disease (specially cyanotic CHD and CCF),
- Chronic lung disease (specially asthma on high dose oral steroids)
- Chronic Kidney disease (specially Nephrotic syndrome)
- Diabetes mellitus
- Cerebrospinal fluid leaks or cochlear implant surgery.
- Asplenia (e.g. Sickle cell disease, congenital, splenectomy)

Immunocompromized children with:
- Congenital immunodeficiency disorders
- HIV/ AIDS
- Immunosuppressive chemo/radio therapy,
- Malignant neoplasms including Leukemia, Lymphoma
- Solid organ transplantation

Prematurity & very Low birth weight (IAP recommendation)

Efficacy: All PCVs have to meet WHO criteria for immunoge-nicity i.e. IgG levels ≥ 0.35 µg/ml for all serotypes collectively and recommended serotype-specific IgG geometric concen-tration ratios. All PCVs are comparably immunogenic with seroprotection rates of >90% following primary doses.

Protective efficacy of PCVs depend on the number of serotypes included in the vaccine and the number of doses given. While all PCVs cover > 70% of serotypes responsible for Invasive pneumococcal disease, coverage is naturally higher with PCV-13 than with PCV-10 by 10-15%.

Protective efficacy of a single dose of PCV13 is estimated as~48%, with two doses as 87% and with 2+1 doses as 100%. One dose catch-up for toddlers showed 83% effectiveness.

In general, Protective efficacy of PCVs is estimated to be ~60% against invasive pneumococcal disease irrespective of serotypes and ~80% p against IPD due to vaccine serotypes, when primary doses are given before 6 months of age. Protective efficacy against invasive disease has been shown to last over 6 years in 78% of cases.

Protective value against Pneumococcal pneumonia is difficult to ascertain due to diagnostic difficulties and hence, usually assessed against any radiological proven pneumonia, which is reported to be ~ 25–35%. Some studies have shown a significant reduction in hospitalizations even due to viral lower respiratory tract infections among PCV vaccinated population,

Protective efficacy for acute otitis media was ~55% in earlier studies using PCV7, though later studies have reported much lower efficacy (15-33%) with PCV7/10 vaccines due to *serotype replacement* i.e. significant reduction in disease due to vaccine serotypes, partly offset by increased contribution of non-vaccine serotypes and other organisms. Interestingly, one PCV-10 trial (synflorix®) showed about 35% protection against otitis media due to 'Non-typeable *H. influenza* attributed to the immune response against the carrier protein used in the vaccine.

Many countries, where PCV is the part of routine immunization, have shown significant reduction in invasive pneumococcal disease not only in vaccinees but also in unvaccinated population due to reduction in nasopharyngeal carriage and transmission of the organism.

Safety: Side-effects are uncommon except local reactions, fever and irritability in ~10% and Gastrointestinal symptoms in ~1% cases. Hypersensitivity reactions, seizures and hypotonic-hyporesponsive episodes have been reported rarely in <0.01% vaccinees.

Serotype replacement: In countries which have introduced PCV in national schedule, studies had shown a rise in the incidence of nasopharyngeal carriage and invasive pneumococcal disease due to serotypes other than those included in the vaccine – a phenomena termed as *serotype replacement*. Surveillance studies from the United States after introduction of PCV7 in their immunization schedule showed a decrease in cases of IPD due to vaccine serotypes and increase in cases due to nonvaccine serotypes Some PCV-10 studies have also shown increase in the otitis media due to serotypes not included in the vaccines.
However, a systemic review by WHO has shown that despite the phenomena of serotype replacement, there is net reduction in IPD cases, including pneumococcal meningitis among under-5 children.

Contraindications include a severe allergic reactions to a prior dose or to any other vaccine, containing diphtheria toxoid (Carrier protein). Safety and efficacy of concurrent administration of PCV13 and PPSV23 is not established and not recommended.

Frequently Asked Questions (FAQs)

1. **Which vaccine is preferable for Pneumococcal immunization in healthy children and why?**

   Only PCVs should be used for immunization of healthy children. PPSV vaccines have no role in immunization of healthy children, used only in high-risk children *in addition to* the PCV.

   All PCVs are almost equally effective and cover > 70% of serotypes responsible for Invasive pneumococcal disease.

However, PCV13 naturally has an edge over PCV10 due to inclusion of more strains with coverage being 10-15% higher than the later vaccine. IAP recommends use of any PCV vaccine (10 or 13) for routine immunization of healthy infants.

2. **Why is PPSV given to high-risk children, in addition to PCV immunization?**

PPSV is a 23-valent vaccine and hence, used to expand serotype coverage against IPD after routine immunization with PCV10/13 vaccine.

3. **Why is it mandatory to give PCV vaccination in a high-risk child despite PPSV vaccination?**

PPSV is poorly immunogenic below 2 years of age, has low immune memory, does not reduce nasopharyngeal carriage and does not provide herd immunity. Hence, PPSV should never be used alone in high-risk children; always to be preceded or succeeded (if already given) with recommended doses of PCV.

4. **Whether PCV and PPSV vaccines can be given simultaneously in high risk children?**

No. safety and efficacy of concurrent administration of PCV-13 and PPV-23 has not been studied, and concurrent administration is not recommended with minimum 8 weeks interval between two vaccines.

5. **Whether it is possible to interchange PCV10 and PCV13 vaccines to complete the series, if necessary?**

Interchangeability between PCV10 and PCV13 is not advisable, but permitted if unavoidable.

6. **Whether PCV vaccine can be given to Preterm and/or low birth weight infants?**

Preterms and Very low birth weight infants have upto 9-fold higher incidence of IPD versus full size babies and IAP recommends PCV immunization to them on priority basis.

7. **Why is a three dose schedule used in NIP as against IAP recommended four dose schedule for routine immunization of healthy children.**

Gold standard for PCV immunization is three primary doses from 6 weeks onwards, preferably two months apart, followed by a booster dose in second year (3p+1 schedule). IAP recommends the same but with primary doses at monthly intervals (6, 10, 14 weeks) to align with existing immunization schedule and minimize number of visits.

However inclusion of PCV in NIS also involves cost considerations without compromise on efficacy and many countries have adopted shortened vaccination schedules.

WHO recommends minimum three doses to all children from 6 weeks of age, either as two primary doses two months apart followed by a booster at 9-15 months (2p+1 schedule) *or* three primary doses without boosters (3p+0). While 2p+1 schedule may leave some infants unprotected between primary and booster doses, second 3p+0 schedule may not provide long-lasting immunity beyond 18 months of age.

India has adopted the 2p+1 schedule (booster at 9 months to align with MR vaccination) as antibody titres achieved with two doses at two-monthly interval are higher than the doses given at monthly intervals and will exceed those achieved with 3p+0 schedule, after the booster dose, providing longer duration of protection.

8. **Which are the newer pneumococcal vaccines under development?**

A 15-valent PCV by *Merck* with two additional serotypes to existing PCV13 (22F and 33F) and a 20-valent PCV by *Pfizer* with seven additional serotypes (8, 10A, 11A, 12F, 15BC, 22F, and 33F) are in pipeline to offset some of the projected replacement serotypes, anticipated to increase after routine PCV-13/10 use.

Key Points

Types: Polysaccharide & Conjugate vaccines

Pneumococcal Conjugate vaccine (PCV):

- **Vaccine:** Polyvalent (PCV10 or PCV13), Single dose, liquid formulation
- **Dose:** IM 0.5 ml/dose (1ml >18 yrs age), over thigh/deltoid
- **Schedule:**
  - *NIS:* Two primary doses at 6 & 14 weeks, Booster at 9 months (Age-limit till 1 year)
  - *IAP:* Three primary doses at 6, 10 & 14 weeks, Booster at 12-15 months
- **Catch-up immunization**: (upto 5 years as per IAP)

  < 6 mo: Three primary doses at 0, 1, 2 mo, Booster at 12–15 mo (6 mo after third dose).

  6-12 mo: Two primary doses at one month interval, Booster in 2nd year.

  12-23 mo: Two primary doses at two month interval, No booster.

  24-59 mo: Two doses at 8-week interval (PCV10) or Single dose of PCV13, No booster.

- **High-risk Cases:** See text.
- **Efficacy:** (10-15% higher with PCV13 than PCV10)

  Invasive disease: ~60-80% as high as 100% after 2+1 doses

  Pneumonia & Otitis Media: ~25-35%,
- **Safety:** Side-effects rare, except Local reaction, mild fever, irritability

  Rarely seizures and Hypotonic–hyporesponsive episodes
- **Contraindications:** None except hypersensitivity to DT containing vaccine

Pneumococcal Polysaccharide Vaccines (PPSV):

Vaccine: Polyvalent (23 serotypes), Single-dose liquid formulation

Dose: IM or SC 0.5 ml/dose (1ml >18 yrs age), over thigh/deltoid

Schedule: Only in high-risk children, to be used alongwith PCV

Single dose after 2 yrs of age, repeat once only after 3-5 yrs

Efficacy: Uncertain, poorly immunogenic before 2 years of age.

Side effects: Rare, no contraindications

Research is also underway to develop serotype-independent pneumococcal vaccines using- a) common protein-based, serotype-independent subunit vaccines, b)

combination (protein vaccine antigens plus polysaccharide conjugates) vaccine, and c) whole-cell vaccine (WCV) comprised of killed *S. pneumoniae* organisms enable the simultaneous presentation of multiple surface protein antigens.

References

1. World Health Organization. Pneumococcal conjugate vaccines. Position paper. Weekly Epid. Record 2019;94: 85-104.
2. Shah A. Pneumococcal vaccines *In:* IAP Guidebook on Immunization 2018-19 - Advisory Committee on Vaccines and Immunization Practices, Indian Academy of Pediatrics, 3rd Edition, New Delhi, Jaypee Brothers 2020; pp 168-206.
3. Shah N K. Rotavirus In: Vashishtha V et al. FAQs on Vaccines and immunization practices. 2nd Edition. .New Delhi, Jaypee Brothers 2015; pp 220-238.

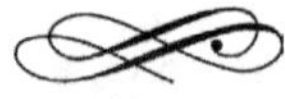

Measles, Mumps & Rubella Vaccines

Vaccines against three common viral illnesses – Measles Mumps and Rubella, are usually available as combination trivalent vaccines (MMR) or bivalent Measles and Rubella vaccine (MR) and hence, discussed here together.

Measles continues to be a significant public health problem in India despite substantial reduction in number of cases and deaths due to expanding immunization coverage and introduction of the second vaccine dose in recent years. India now aims to eliminate measles with intensified immunization programs. Current coverage with first dose of measles containing vaccines in India is about 81%, with considerable state-wise differences.

Rubella *per se* is a mild exanthematous illness but maternal infection in the first trimester may lead to serious health problems in the fetus i.e. Congenital Rubella syndrome (CRS). Currently, India contributes to over one-third of CRS cases, born globally. While Rubella vaccination coverage has been expanding in recent years after introduction of MR vaccine in the NIS, it is still far from satisfactory i.e. merely ~ 24%. Poor Rubella coverage may also be counterproductive by shifting the age-epidemiology of disease from early childhood to older reproductive years with paradoxically higher risk of CRS.

Although generally considered as least of three devils in MMR triology, estimated disease burden of Mumps in India is expected to higher than Rubella, and now even than Measles. Unlike other two diseases, Mumps has the potential to cause complications in both – in the affected child e.g. Orchitis, aseptic meningitis, pancreatitis etc, as well as in unborn fetus following maternal infection e.g. aqueductal stenosis leading to congenital hydrocephalus.

Epidemiology: All three viruses – Measles, Mumps and Rubella, are RNA viruses with only one known serotype for each and spread as droplet infection from a clinical or subclinical case.

Measles predominantly affects the preschool children and is highly contagious with a secondary attack rate of ~80%. Outbreaks are common in winter or spring season. Natural infection usually leads to life-long immunity.

Rubella is usually acquired in the school-age and infection remains unnoticed with asymptomatic or mild self-limiting illness. About 80% of Indian population is infected by late adolescence with life-long immunity. However, 20-30% of women in reproductive age remain susceptible for rubella infection during pregnancy with consequent risk of fetal infection. CRS occurs only if the mother is infected during first trimester.

Mumps is more common in 5-9 year age group, though no age is immune except infants below 6 months of age due to presence of maternal antibodies. Outbreaks are common in late winter or spring season. Life-long immunity develops after clinical/subclinical attack or immunization.

Vaccine: Trivalent MMR vaccine is the most commonly used vaccine world-wide against three viruses, followed by Bivalent MR vaccine. A quadrivalent vaccine including Varicella i.e. MMRV (Priorix tetra®), is also available. Stand-alone Rubella vaccine is available but rarely used, stand-alone Mumps vaccine was never available and stand-alone measles vaccine has been withdrawn from India, replaced with MR vaccine.

All Measles containing vaccines (MR/MMR) are live attenuated vaccines derived from different strains of respective viruses, grown on human diploid cells or purified chick embryo cells. Commonly used strains include *Edmonston Zagreb* and *Schwarz* strains for Measles, *Leningrad-Zagreb* or *Urabe AM9* strains for Mumps and *Wister RA 27/3* strain for Rubella virus. MMRV contains additional *Oka* strain of varicella.

Content & storage: All MR/MMR vaccines (including MMRV) are Freeze-dried vaccines, supplied as single-dose or multi-dose vials with distilled water as diluents, to be reconstituted before use. Post-reconstitution, each single dose (0.5 ml) of vaccine contains, depending on the constituents, not less than 1000 $CCID_{50}$ of Measles virus, 1000 $CCID_{50}$ of Rubella virus and 5000 $CCID_{50}$ of Mumps virus.

All these vaccines must be stored at 2–8°C. Reconstituted vaccines are light and heat labile, to be kept at 2–8°C away from light and must be used within 3-6 hours. These vaccines do not contain any preservative and hence, highly susceptible to contamination after reconstitution, specially when multi-dose vials are used. Severe and sometimes fatal reactions, e.g. toxic-shock syndrome, have been reported with use of reconstituted vaccines beyond 3–6 hours.

Diluent may be stored at room temperature and should never be frozen. Only the diluent supplied with specific vaccine must be used for reconstitution, as it is free from preservatives or other antiviral substances which might inactivate the vaccine. Commonly available *"Water for injections"* must not be used for this purpose.

Dose & administration: Irrespective of the composition, dose of all these vaccines is 0.5 ml subcutaneously, to be given preferably over the upper arm or anterolateral thigh.

Immunization schedule: In NIS, *Two doses of MR Vaccine are recommended at 9-12 months and at 16-24 months.* As transplacental antibody titers may persist till 6–8 months of age, measles vaccination is not recommended before 9 months of age, except during outbreaks when it may be given from 6 months onwards. However, any baby, who has received measles vaccine before 9 months should receive an additional dose at 9 months to ensure adequate seroconversion. *For catch-up immunization Under NIS, MR is given only till 5 years of age with two doses at least at 4 weeks interval.*

IAP recommends use of MMR, instead of MR vaccine, to be given as three doses at 9 months, 15 months and 4-6 years (or any time after 4 weeks of second dose) with following rationale - a) Mumps is a common but under-reported disease in India with significant morbidity including the risk to unborn fetus in pregnancy, b) Single vaccine protects against three common viral illnesses with fairly adequate seroconversion rates for all components.

Unlike MR, third dose of MMR at 4-6 years is recommended as antibody titers against mumps are known to decline over years, leaving the child relatively unprotected at an older age. Otherwise, two doses of measles and single dose of Rubella provide sufficient long-term protection. MMRV can be used as third dose at 4-6 years.

Catch-up Immunization after first year of age involves two doses of MMR vaccines at least four weeks apart, with no upper age limit. However, pregnancy should be excluded before vaccination in adolescent girls, due to potentially teratogenic risk of CRS. Combination MMRV vaccine cannot be used beyond 12 years of age.

Efficacy: *Seroconversion rate against measles* after any measles containing vaccine depends on the age of vaccination i.e. ~80-85% at 9 months and > 95% at or after 12 months of age. Although antibody titers wane over the years, measles-specific cellular immunity persists to provide lifelong protection and secondary vaccine failures are rare after two doses of measles containing vaccine, with at least one dose after 12 months of age.

Seroconversion rate against Rubella is even better following any rubella containing vaccine i.e. 95%. When given below 12 months and 99% above 12 months. Thus, almost all vaccinated infants are protected for Rubella after the second dose of MR/MMR. Although antibody titers decline with time, sufficient time is available for an anamnestic response following Rubella exposure due to long incubation period of disease (14-21 days), to allow life-long protection even in cases with sub-optimal titers.

Seroconversion rates against mumps following MMR vaccination is initially >90% but antibody titers decline with time. Actual protective efficacy of the mumps component of MMR is ~78% with single dose and 88% with two doses. Outbreaks have been reported in previously vaccinated populations with sub-optimal titers and hence, minimum two doses are needed for durable protection with second dose at about 5-6 years, as recommended by IAP.

Efficacy of MMRV is comparable to MMR and Varicella vaccines given separately.

Safety: MR/MMR vaccines are safe, except mild local reactions, transient morbilliform rash with mild fever after 7-12 days in 2-5% and Thrombocytopenic purpura after first week in 1:30000 vaccinees. Transient immunosuppression for 3-4 weeks is common after Measles vaccination.

Measles vaccine has been implicated in some post-vaccination deaths, due to inadequate aseptic precautions. These vaccines do not contain any preservative and should be used within 4-6 hours of reconstitution. Bacterial contamination of multi-dose vials may lead to development of Toxic-shock syndrome. Few deaths due to inadvertent use of wrong diluents e.g. succinylcholine, have also been reported.

Rubella/Rubella-containing vaccines apart from the side-effects as above, are also known to cause transient arthralgia/arthritis after 1-3 weeks in about 10-25% adolescent and adult female vaccinees, though rarely in children or older males..

Mumps-containing vaccines are known to cause high fever after 7-12 days, febrile seizures, Transient Parotitis and mild aseptic meningitis after 2–3 weeks.

Side-effects e.g. fever, rash and febrile seizures are more common with MMRV, specially in younger children of 12-23 months not primed with Measles vaccine earlier and hence, MMRV should be used only for third dose at 4-6 years of age.

Although implicated in the past, there is no data to support causal relationship between MR/MMR vaccine and Guillain Barre Syndrome, Autism and Inflammatory bowel diseases. Very rarely, Encephalitis including subacute sclerosing panencephalitis (SSPE) has been reported following measles vaccination (1/million doses) though the causal association is not proven. There is no reported instance of the transmission of the vaccine virus to the contacts.

Contraindications for MR/MMR vaccines include:

- *Severe Immunodeficiency states.* Vaccine may be administered to those with HIV infection unless severely immunocompromised, as the benefits outweigh the risks.

- *Severe egg allergy,* if an MR/MMR vaccine derived from chick embryo is used.

- *Active Tuberculosis:* Measles vaccine induces a transient state of immunosuppression, like the natural disease. Hence, it should be deferred in cases with active

Tuberculosis, till antitubercular therapy has been given for 4–6 weeks. For the same reason, it should not be given along with BCG or other vaccines, to ensure uptake of other vaccines.

- *Pregnancy:* Rubella-containing vaccines are contraindicated in pregnancy and Pregnancy should be avoided for 3 months after vaccination. However, babies born to accidentally vaccinated women during pregnancy have not shown increased risk of congenital malformations and medical termination of pregnancy in these cases is not warranted.

- *Thromobocytopenic purpura* or history of thrombocytopenic purpura following previous dose of measles/ MMR vaccine. In such cases, it should be given with after weighing risks versus benefits.

- *Hypersensitivity reaction* to previous dose or neomycin as some vaccines may contain the traces of neomycin.

Frequently Asked Questions (FAQs)

1. **Why is MR vaccine used in NIS rather than MMR, despite significant disease burden in Indian population?**

    MR rather than MMR has been included in the National immunization schedule considering that– a) disability component of mumps is not a serious public health problem, and b) Addition of mumps component would result in the substantial increase in the cost (2-3 times) without commensurate public health benefits.

2. **Then, why does IAP recommends MMR instead of MR?**

    IAP recommends MMR instead of MR vaccine as it considers that - a) Mumps is a common but largely under-reported disease in India, with b) significant morbidity, including the risk to pregnant woman in terms of fetal damage e.g. aqueductal stenosis. Not including Mumps component with MR vaccination will be a missed opportunity to attack a common disease with significant morbidity. Further, MR is not available commercially at present.

3. Why is MR vaccine given at 9 months of age, when immunogenicity is better beyond infancy?

MR vaccination at 9 months is an epidemiological compulsion despite lower seroconversion rates below 12 months of age (80-85% *vs* > 95%) due to the need for early protection as significant proportion of measles cases in India occur in late infancy. Second dose of MR/MMR at 12-15 months covers this immunogenicity deficit of first 9-month dose.

WHO recommends that in countries with low rates of transmission first dose of Measles vaccine be given at 12 months to take advantage of better seroconversion rates.

4. Why does IAP recommend a third dose of MMR at 4-6 years?

Two doses of measles vaccine and one dose of rubella vaccine suffice for long term protection. However, two doses of mumps-containing vaccine may not be as effective as antibody titers decline significantly over time. Hence, the Third dose of MMR at 4-6 years age has been added to prevent mumps outbreaks in the older children and adolescents.

In a child above 12 months, who has not received MR/MMR at 9 months, only two doses of MMR at 8 weeks interval are sufficient with second dose mainly to protect children who fail to seroconvert against primarily mumps and less commonly against rubella by the first dose (primary vaccine failures).

5. Whether combined MMRV vaccine can be used instead of MMR and Varicella vaccines given separately?

While MMR+V (separately) and MMRV (combination) have shown comparable seroconversion rates for all four antigens, side-effects e.g. fever, rash and febrile seizures are more common with MMRV in younger children of 12-23 months, specially in those who have not been primed earlier with Measles vaccine.

Hence, IAP recommends that the MMR and varicella vaccines must be given separately (MMR+V) at 15 months age, though either the same (MMR+V) or MMRV can be offered at 4-6 years of age as per parental preference.

For catch-up immunization of older children above 48 months, not immunized earlier with MMR and varicella vaccines, both options are open with either two doses of MMRV or MMR + V, given 6-12 weeks apart. It is to be noted that MMRV is licensed only till 12 yrs of age and anyone older, who needs protection from these diseases should get MMR and varicella vaccines as separate shots.

6. **Does a child need to be vaccinated if s/he has past history of Measles?**

Yes, as many viral illnesses mimic measles and the diagnosis cannot be foolproof in most cases. All children with history of measles need two doses of MR/MMR as per age-wise /catch-up recommendations.

7. **What should be done is a child comes for MR/MMR immunization late, after infancy?**

Catch-up Immunization after first year of age involves only two doses of MMR vaccines at least four weeks apart, with no upper age limit. However, pregnancy should be excluded before vaccination in adolescent girls, due to potentially teratogenic risk of CRS. Under NIS, MR is given only upto 5 years of age.

8. **If a child has received the MR vaccine before 9 months of age, is it necessary to repeat the vaccine later?**

Yes. MR vaccine can be given as early as 6 months during outbreaks. However, the immunogenicity of this early dose in low (~60%) due to presence of maternal antibodies and all such cases should receive regular doses at 9 month and 12-15 months.

9. **Why is it necessary to immunize male children against rubella?**

   If a male child develops rubella, he may infect other contacts e.g. unimmunized pregnant women in the family with potential risk of CRS. Hence, it is important that everyone, including males, are protected against rubella to prevent rubella transmission and outbreaks.

10. **Can MR and JE vaccine be given together in Routine Immunization?**

    Yes, In JE endemic districts, both MR and JE vaccine are given together in NIS at the same time but on different arms. However, if these vaccines couldn't be given on the same day, a minimum gap of 4 weeks has to be maintained as a standard practice between any two live vaccines.

11. **Whether measles vaccine can be given in an HIV-infected child?**

    MR/MMR are live vaccines, contraindicated in symptomatic HIV infected children or those with severe immunosuppression. However, it may be given to asymptomatic cases without significant immunosuppression, as the benefits outweigh the risks. Immunogenicity may be lower in these cases. Interestingly, studies have shown better seroconversion rates in HIV infected children following measles vaccination at 6 months as compared to 9 months, due to progressive immunodeficiency with age.

12. **Can MR/MMR vaccine be used for post-exposure prophylaxis for Measles?**

    Administration of the vaccine within two days of exposure protects against or modifies the severity of clinical disease.

13. **What is follow-up MR campaign?**

    India conducted a Measles-rubella (MR) vaccination campaign in during 2017-2019 to strengthen the immunization coverage for these two diseases with an aim to eliminate measles and control Congenital rubella syndrome by 2020. It aimed to cover all children from 9 months to 15 years of age with a single dose of MR vaccine, to be given in schools, community centers and health facilities, irrespective of previous vaccination status. Immediately after the completion of campaign, MR vaccine replaced the stand-alone measles vaccine in routine NIS.

Measles-Rubella Follow-up Campaign is a follow-up mass vaccination campaign organized as a periodic event, to be conducted every 3–5 years, depending on the accumulation of susceptible cohorts based on the surveillance data. It aims to target children born after the last campaign to achieve and sustain a high level of population immunity.

Key Points

- **Vaccine:** Live attenuated stand-alone (Rubella) or Combination vaccines (MR, MMR, MMRV)

- **Contents:** All Freeze-dried vaccines, supplied with diluents. Use within 6 hrs of reconstitution.

- **Dose:** SC 0.5 ml/dose (1ml >18 yrs age), over Thigh/deltoid region

- **Schedule:**

  - *NIS:* Total Two doses of MR vaccine at 9 mo and 12-15 mo

  - *IAP:* Total Three doses of MMR Vaccine at 9 mo, 15 mo and 4-6 yr

- **Catch-up immunization:** No upper age limit (Upto 5 years in NIS)

  Two doses of MR/MMR at minimum 4 weeks interval.

- **Efficacy:** Measles 80-95%, Rubella 95-99% Mumps (88-90%)

- **Safety:** Side-effects are rare, except -

  - Local, Fever, Rash, Purpura, SSPE? (due to Measles component)

  - Arthralgia/Arthritis (due to Rubella component)

  - Parotitis or Aseptic meningitis (due to Mumps component)

  - Toxic shock syndrome due to contamination of reconstituted vaccine

- **Contraindications:** Severe Immunodeficiency, Active Tuberculosis, severe egg allergy, Pregnancy.

References

1. World Health Organization. Measles vaccines Position paper: Weekly Epid. Record 2017;92:205-228.
2. World Health Organization. Rubella vaccines: Position paper: Weekly Epid. Record 2011;86:301-316
3. World Health Organization. Mumps vaccines. Position paper: Weekly Epid. Record 2007;82: 49-60
4. Ministry of Health and Welfare, Govt. of India. National operational guideline for introduction of Measles-Rubella vaccine 2017.
5. Shah A. Measles, Mumps and Rubella vaccines: *In:* IAP Guidebook on Immunization 2018-19 - Advisory Committee on Vaccines and Immunization Practices, Indian Academy of Pediatrics, 3rd.
6. Edition, New Delhi, Jaypee Brothers 2020; pp 227-245. Prajapati BS. Measles mumps and Rubella *In:* Vashishtha V et al. FAQs on Vaccines and immunization practices. 2nd Edition. New Delhi, Jaypee Brothers 2015; pp 195-207.
7. Vashishtha VM et al. IAP Position Paper on Burden of Mumps in India and Vaccination Strategies Indian Pediatrics 2015;52; 505-514.

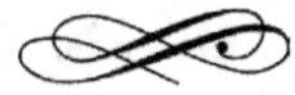

Japanese Encephalitis Vaccines

Japanese encephalitis (JE) is a major public health problem with seasonal outbreaks in different parts of country, specially North India. Since the first reported case from Vellore in 1955, disease is now endemic in twelve states including Uttar pradesh, West Bengal, Bihar, Karnataka, Tamil Nadu, Andhra pradesh, Assam, Manipur and Goa.

JE is a leading cause of viral encephalitis in children and adolescents with high case fatality rate of ~20-30% and neurological sequelae in other 30-40% cases. However, Subclinical infections are 250-1000 times more common than clinical cases.

Epidemiology: JE virus is an RNA virus, transmitted by *Culex* mosquito and outbreaks are common in monsoon or post-monsoon season though sporadic cases occur throughout the year. Risk is higher in children though recent years have seen rising incidence in adults due to epidemiological shift following increasing immunization coverage in children.

Vaccine: Currently, three JE vaccines are licensed in India—a *live attenuated vaccine* derived from SA14-14-2 strain and two *inactivated vero-cell culture derived vaccines* from different strains - SA14-14-2 strain (JEEV®) and 825146XY strain from Kolar, India (JENVAC®)

Of these, the live attenuated SA14-14-2 JE vaccine, imported from China (Chengdu Institute of Biological Products) is exclusively used in the national immunization program. Both inactivated vaccines are produced in India and are commercially available.

Other inactivated (IXIARO®), or live attenuated recombinant vaccines (IMOJEV®) from SA14-14-2 strains are also available but not licensed in India at present.

Contents & Storage: Live attenuated JE vaccine, used in NIS, is a *lyophilized vaccine* which needs to be reconstituted before use. It is relatively heat stable and can be stored at 37°C for 7–10 days, at room temperature for 4 months and at 2–8°C for at least 1.5 years till expiry.

Both commercially available inactivated vaccines are single dose 0.5 ml (6 µg) liquid formulations, which must be stored at 2–8°C.

Dosage & Administration: Live attenuated vaccine is given subcutaneously as 0.5 ml/dose over left upper arm. *Inactivated vaccines* are given 0.5 ml intramuscularly over anterolateral thigh or deltoid region. However, the dose of inactivated JEEV® in children below 3 years is half i.e. 0.25 ml/dose.

Immunization Schedule: Under NIS, JE vaccine is given only in notified endemic districts of country, as two doses at 9-12 months (with MR-1 vaccine) and 16-24 months (with DPT Booster and MR-2 doses) over the left upper arm.

Commercially available Inactivated vaccines are given as two doses, one month apart after one year of age.

Catch-up immunization is recommended up to 15 years of age. However, mass vaccination of children has led to an upward epidemiological shift in age with rising numbers of adult JE cases in some endemic regions. Consequently, IAP has raised the upper age limit for JE immunization from 15 to 18 years. Some endemic states e.g. Assam, conduct special drives to immunize adults >15 years in high-endemic regions.

Efficacy: A neutralization antibody titer of > 1:10 is considered as a correlate of protection for JR vaccines.

Studies from china and Nepal have shown *protective efficacy* of >80% with single dose and >95% with two doses of live vaccines. In India, till recently only single dose was used with lower seroconversion rate of ~70% after 28 days and protective efficacy of 40-70% for one year. Lower efficacy in Indian children was perhaps due to the presence of neutralizing antibodies in over 45% cases before vaccination. Government of India has introduced two-dose schedule in endemic districts since 2013 and field results for protective efficacy of two-dose schedule are awaited.

Reported seroconversion rates after two doses of inactivated vaccines are 56.3% on day 28 (92.4% on day 56) with JEEV vaccine and 93.1% on day 28 (96.9% on day 56) with JENVAC vaccine. While seroconversion rates are higher with JENVAC, titres decline rapidly. Need for a booster dose is not yet established.

Safety: Live attenuated vaccine used in NIS is very safe except transient fever in 5–10% and local reactions, rash or irritability in 1–3%. No hypersensitivity reactions or acute encephalitis have been reported. Inactivated vaccines are equally safe.

Contraindications are none but may be deferred during acute severe febrile illness.

Frequently Asked Questions (FAQs)

1. **Whether JE vaccination is a part of National Immunization schedule?**

    JE vaccination is a part of national Immunization schedule since 2006 but only in notified endemic districts (Currently covering 268 districts).

2. **Whether JE vaccine is available in private sector?**

    Live JE vaccine is only for use under NIS. However. inactivated vaccines are available commercially.

3. **What should be the JE immunization plan for a 15 month old child, who had missed the first dose at 9 months?**

    First dose should be given at first contact and the second dose after 3 months of the first dose.

4. **Whether any booster dose is required for JE vaccine?**

    Boosters are not recommended for live attenuated vaccine used in NIS as protection lasts for over 5 years even with single dose. Further, the boosting is expected in endemic regions due to natural sub-clinical infections.

    While seroconversion rates are high even with inactivated JE vaccines, titres decline rapidly and booster doses have been recommended in some countries. However, the need and timing for a booster dose with inactivated vaccines available in India is not yet determined.

5. **Whether JE vaccine can be given as post-exposure prophylaxis or during outbreaks?**

    Japanese encephalitis vaccine should not be used as an *outbreak response vaccine*, recommended for universal immunization of children living in endemic regions.

6. **Whether JE vaccination is also recommended for adults living in endemic regions?**

    Upper age limit for catch-up JE immunization in endemic regions is 15 years (18 years as per IAP) as older population is expected to be protected due to sub-clinical natural infections. However, an epidemiological shift has been observed in some endemic regions due to increasing immunization coverage of children with rising incidence of disease in adults. Hence, some states e.g. Assam have begin to conduct special immunization activities for JE vaccination in adolescents and adults above 15 years of age in selected severely affected districts.

7. What are recommendations for JE vaccination to travellers?

It is recommended for travellers only if they expect to stay for at least 4 weeks in rural areas of endemic regions during the JE season.

8. Whether JE vaccine can be given with other vaccines?

Yes. In fact under NIS, first dose of JE vaccine is recommended with MR-1 vaccine and second dose with MR-2 and DPT booster. However, all co-administered vaccines must be given at different sites conventionally- JE vaccine on left upper arm, MR1/2 on Right upper arm and DPT on antero-lateral side of mid-thigh.

Key points

- **Vaccine:** Live attenuated (used under NIS) and Inactivated vaccines (available commercially)

- **Dose:** Live attenuated vaccine: SC 0.5 ml

  Inactivated vaccine: IM 0.5 ml (0.25 ml for JEEV <3 yrs of age)

- **Immunization Schedule:**

  - NIS *(Live attenuated vaccine, only in endemic districts)*
    Two doses at 9 -12 months & 16-24 months of age

  - Commercial Inactivated vaccine
    Two doses at one month interval

- **Catch-up immunization:** 15 years (NIS), 18 years (IAP)

- **Efficacy:** Live attenuated vaccine: 40-70% after single dose
  (Not established with two doses)
  Inactivated vaccine: >90% after two doses

- **Safety:** Side-effects uncommon, except mild fever and local reaction

- **Contraindications** none, defer during acute severe febrile illness.

References

1. World Health Organization. Japanese encephalitis vaccines. Position paper.: Weekly Epid. Record 2015;90: 69-88.
2. Guduru VK. Japanese Encephalitis Vaccines: *In*: IAP Guidebook on Immunization 2018-19 - Advisory Committee on Vaccines and Immunization Practices, Indian Academy of Pediatrics, 3rd Edition, New Delhi, Jaypee Brothers 2020; pp 333-351.
3. Vashishtha VM Japanese Encephalitis *In:* Vashishtha V et al. FAQs on Vaccines and immunization practices. 2nd Edition. .New Delhi, Jaypee Brothers 2015; pp 254-267.
4. Ministry of Health and Family Welfare, Government of India. Control of Japanese Encephalitis. Operational Guide Japanese Encephalitis Vaccination in India. 2010; pp. 13-5.

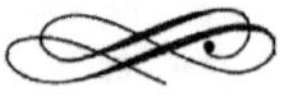

Section

III

Additional Recommended vaccines
(Indian Academy of Pediatrics)

Enteric fever is one of the leading causes of prolonged pyrexia in children. Overall disease burden, emergence of extensive drug resistance and significant case fatality rate of 1-4% justifies the need for typhoid vaccination and IAP has strongly recommended to include typhoid vaccine in NIS.

Epidemiology: *S. typhi* is a gram-negative organism with three major antigens (O, H, Vi) and over 80 phagetypes. Virulence is mainly determined by Vi (Virulence) antigen. Reservoir of infection is a case or asymptomatic carrier and infection is transmitted feco-orally. Typhoid fever is more common in school-age children and adolescents, during rainy season and in urban slums due to unhygienic living conditions.

Vaccines: Currently, two types of typhoid vaccines are available in India, both active against the virulent (Vi) antigen - a) Vi polysaccharide vaccine (TPSV) and (b) Vi-polysaccharide conjugate vaccine (TCV), using a carrier protein to boost its immunogenicity.

Early generation whole cell inactivated typhoid vaccines have been withdrawn due to higher side effects. A Live Attenuated (Ty21a) vaccine is also available in some countries but not in India and hence, not discussed here

16.1: TYPHOID POLYSACCHARIDE VACCINE (TPSV)

TPSV contains highly purified fraction of Vi-capsular poly-saccharide antigen. Being a pure polysaccharide vaccine, it is poorly immunogenic, specially in children below 2 years of age and does not produce immunological memory.

Contents & storage: Each dose contains 25 μg of purified polysaccharide in 0.5 ml of phenolic isotonic buffer, supplied as single dose ampoule or vial and to be stored at 2-8°C.

Dosage & administration: TPSV can be used only in children above 2 years, given as 0.5 ml/dose intramuscularly or deep subcutaneously over thigh or deltoid region.

Immunization Schedule: Typhoid vaccination is not included in NIS. IAP recommends it to all healthy children, but using a conjugate vaccine (discussed later) rather than TPSV due to better immunogenicity and longer duration of protection.

However, TPSV can be considered for routine immunization in individuals aged 2 years and older with a single dose, to be repeated every three years. Catch-up vaccination is recommended up to 18 years.

Efficacy: Serological correlate of protection for typhoid vaccines is not well established, though Anti-Vi antibodies titer of ≥ 1 μg/ml or four-fold rise in titers are generally acceptable. Antibodies titer of ≥ 4.3 μg/ml are usually considered as adequate to sustain the protection for 4 years.

While Seroconversion rate with TPSV is >90%, protective efficacy in the field trials has been reported as only ~55–70% for 2–3 years, which drops further over time, necessitating re-vaccination every 3 years. *Repeat dose is not a booster dose* as immunological response to unconjugated Vi-PS is T-cell independent without development of immune memory. Repeated vaccinations are not reported to cause hyporesponsiveness.

Interestingly, a study from Kolkata slums has shown the *herd protection* against Typhoid in 44% in unvaccinated children in the vaccinated cluster.

Safety: Side-effects are rare, except local pain and erythema. Vaccine does not interfere with interpretation of Widal test.

Contraindications: None, except past history of hypersensitivity to the vaccine. It can be safely given in immunocompromised children.

16.2: TYPHOID CONJUGATE VACCINE (TCV)

Presently, four Typhoid Conjugate Vaccine against Vi polysaccharide antigen are licensed in India - three conjugated with Tetanus toxoid (*Pedatyph®, Zyvac-TCV®, Typbar-TCV®*) and one conjugated with detoxified diphtheria toxin CRM197 (Typhibev®).

Contents & storage: All TCV contain 25µg conjugated Vi antigen suspended in 0.5 ml of isotonic saline, except Pedityph®, which contains only 5 µg. These vaccines need to be stored at 2-8°C and some of them have vaccine vial monitor to ensure proper storage.

Dosage & administration: TCVs are given as 0.5 ml/dose, intramuscularly or deep subcutaneously over deltoid or thigh region.

Immunization Schedule: While not included in NIS, IAP recommends a single dose of TCV vaccine at 6-9 months of age as part of routine immunization to all infants. Booster dose is no longer recommended. TCV can be clubbed with MMR vaccine, if given after 9 months.

Catch-up vaccination is recommended up to 18 years of age. IAP also recommends a single dose of TCV to a child who has received TPSV earlier, at least 4 weeks after TPSV.

Efficacy: Reported seroconversion rate after 42 days of TCV is > 98% in children vaccinated above 6 months of age. Although antibody titers wane over time, all vaccinees continue to be protected for up to 3-5 years and Immunity is further boosted due to subsequent sub-clinical natural infections.

WHO position paper, 2018, has remarked that the evidence about efficacy of low-dose (5 µg) TCV i.e. Pediatyph® is limited. IAP does not recommend use of this low-dose vaccine at present.

Safety: All TCV vaccines are safe except fever and local reactions at injection site. Fever is more common in younger children.

Frequently Asked Questions (FAQs)

1. **Why is TCV preferred over TPSV for routine immunization?**

   TCVs are preferred over TPV due to better immuno-genicity (>98% vs 90%), better protective value (85% vs <70%) and longer duration of protection (3-5 yr vs 2-3 yrs) apart from the fact that TPSVs cannot be used in children below 2 years due to poor immunogenicity of polysaccharide vaccines. Further, TPSVs do not induce T-cell dependent immunological memory with poor anamnestic response on re-exposure.

2. **Whether a booster dose can be used to potentiate the immune response of TPSV, if TCV is not given?**

   TPSV is a polysaccharide vaccine, does not produce immunological memory and booster dose is of no use in this case.

3. **Why does IAP recommend only a single dose of TCV for primary vaccination though higher antibody titers have been demonstrated with two-dose schedule?**

   Although geometric mean antibody titers (GMTs) achieved with single dose are marginally lower than those with two doses, studies have shown comparable seroconversion rate of >80-100% with both schedules. Further, there was no significant difference in the seroprotection rate and protective value even after 2-3 years, which continue to exceed >85%. Hence, currently, only one primary dose is recommended.

4. **Why is a booster dose not recommended after TCV vaccines even when antibody titers are known to wane after 3-5 years?**

   A single dose of the TCV vaccine after 6 months of age provides a reasonably good GMTs and seroconversion rate in most of the vaccinees, lasting for at least 3 years after vaccination. Later, frequent sub-clinical natural infections in older children lead to immunological boosting and obviate the need of further boosters.

5. **Why does IAP not recommend use of Pediatyph® at present?**

   Antibody titers depend on the antigenic dose. Pedatyph contains only 5 µg of antigen *versus* 25 µg in other licensed TCVs. Studies have shown higher GMT levels following vaccination with high-antigen TCVs than the low-antigen TCV. While protective antibody titers are not well established for these vaccines and even lower GMT values achieved after low-antigen Pediatyph might be protective, WHO position paper 2018 has remarked that the body of evidence for the 5 µg vaccine (Pediatyph®) is limited. IAP too does not recommend this low-dose vaccine at present, despite being licensed in India.

6. **Whether Typhoid vaccination prevents against Paratyphoid fever?**

   No. *Salmonella enterica* serovars paratyphi A, B and rarely C, cause a disease termed as Paratyphoid fever, which may be clinically indistinguishable from typhoid fever. However, Vi locus is absent from *S. paratyphi* A and B and hence, Vi polysaccharide vaccines do not protect against paratyphoid fever.

7. **Whether a child with history of confirmed Typhoid fever needs to be vaccinated.?**

   Yes. A child with history of suspected or confirmed enteric fever must be vaccinated 4 weeks after recovery if he/she has not received the vaccine in the past 3 years.

8. Whether Typhoid vaccination affects Widal test reports?

No. Widal test assesses agglutinin titers against H and O typhoid antigens, while Typhoid vaccines use purified Vi antigen. Hence, current typhoid vaccines do not interfere with interpretation of Widal test, unlike earlier generation whole cell inactivated typhoid vaccines.

Key Points
Types: Conjugate vaccine (TCV) and Polysaccharide vaccine (TPSV)

TCV vaccine:

- **Vaccine:** Conjugate (Vi) vaccine, liquid formulation
- **Dose:** IM 0.5 ml/dose (1ml >18 yrs age), over thigh/deltoid
- **Schedule** (Not included in NIS):
  - Single dose at 6-9 months of age, No booster
- **Catch-up immunization:** Upto 18 years
- **Efficacy:** >98% for 3-5 years, Protective efficacy 55-70% for 2-3 yrs
- **Safety:** Side-effects rare, except Local reaction, fever
- **Contraindications:** None, except hypersensitivity to vaccine constituents

TPSV vaccine:

- **Vaccine:** Polysaccharide (Vi) vaccine, liquid formulation
- **Dose:** IM/SC 0.5 ml/dose over thigh/deltoid region
- **Schedule:** Not included in NIS.
  - Single dose at 2 years of age, repeated 3 years (If TCV is not feasible)
- **Catch-up vaccination:** Upto 18 years
- **Efficacy:** Seroconversion rate >90%, Protective efficacy 55-70% for 2-3 yrs
- **Safety:** Side-effects rare except fever and local reactions.
- **Contraindications:** None, except hypersensitivity to previous dose.

References

1. World Health Organization. Typhoid vaccines: Position paper. Weekly Epid. Record 2018;93:153-172.
2. Guduru VK. Typhoid Vaccines: *In:* IAP Guidebook on Immunization 2018-19 - Advisory Committee on Vaccines and Immunization Practices, Indian Academy of Pediatrics, 3rd Edition, New Delhi, Jaypee Brothers 2020; pp 278-301.
3. Kalra A et al. Typhoid *In:* Vashishtha V et al. FAQs on Vaccines and immunization practices. 2nd Edition. .New Delhi, Jaypee Brothers 2015; pp 208-214.

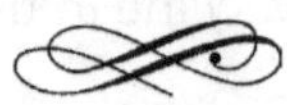

Hepatitis A (HAV) is the common cause of jaundice in India, though clinical disease is generally mild and self-limiting. Severity of the disease increases with age. Complications are rare though acute hepatic failure following HAV infection is being increasingly observed even in children.

Epidemiology: HAV is a single-stranded RNA Picornavirus with only one serotype but multiple genotypes. It is excreted in stools of a clinical or subclinical case and transmitted via the feco-oral route by ingestion of contaminated water/food. Focal outbreaks are common in summer and rainy season, specially in slums due to poor sanitary conditions. Older children and adults often acquire natural immunity following recurrent infections in childhood. Risk of the disease among unvaccinated population increases paradoxically as sanitary conditions improve, due to lesser likelihood of natural infections. In India, ~ 30-40% of adolescents and adults are seronegative, specially those from higher socioeconomic class.

Vaccines: Currently, Two types of HAV vaccines are available in India—

a) Formalin *inactivated vaccines* derived from HM 175/GBM grown on MRC5 human diploid cell lines or RG-SB strain harvested from disrupted MRC-5 cells, and

b) *Live attenuated vaccine,* derived from the H2 strain attenuated after serial passage in Human Diploid Cell.

HAV vaccine is also available in combination with Hepatitis B vaccine (Twinrix®) or typhoid Vi-polysaccharide vaccine (later one not available in India).

Contents & Storage: Inactivated vaccines are available in different formulations for children (0.5 ml) and adults (1.0 ml). Live attenuated vaccine is a freeze-dried vaccine, supplied with diluent. All vaccines need to be stored at 2–8°C.

Dosage & Administration: Inactivated vaccines are given Intramuscularly as 0.5 ml in children and 1.0 ml in adults above 19 years of age. Live attenuated vaccine is given subcutaneously 0.5 ml, irrespective of the age.

Immunization Schedule: HAV vaccines are currently not included in NIS.

All HAV vaccines are licensed for use only in children above 12 months. IAP recommends two doses of Inactivated HAV vaccine 6–18 months apart, starting from 12 to 23 months of age *or* a single dose of Live HAV Vaccine in children.

Catch-up immunization may be given at any age. However, IAP recommends pre-vaccination screening for HAV antibodies in children >10 years, due to higher chance of natural infection and >50% seropositivity by this age.

Combined HAV and HBV vaccine may be used in three-dose schedule (0, 1, 6 months), for catch-up immunization in previously HBV-unimmunized children.

Efficacy: Considering an antibody titer of >20 mI U/ml as the correlate of seroprotection, two doses of inactivated HAV vaccine provide > 90–95% seroprotection for over 10 years. However, the real-life protective efficacy is life-long due to anamnestic response following natural infections with median predicted duration of protection estimated as ~45 years. No boosters are recommended in immunocompetent population. Efficacy is lower in the elderly *or* in those with chronic liver disease *or* immunocompromised states.

Studies have shown higher antibody titers after two doses than after a single dose of inactivated vaccine, though single dose is similarly efficacious, less expensive and provides effective post-exposure prophylaxis against hepatitis A, when given within 2 weeks of exposure. In high-risk cases for hepatitis A, a two-dose vaccination schedule is preferred.

Live HAV vaccine has been shown to have better and longer protective efficacy of upto 100% for pre-exposure prophylaxis and 95% for post-exposure prophylaxis. Anti-HAV antibodies have been detected in 72–88% of the vaccines even 15 years after vaccination. However, it does not provide post-exposure protection during the outbreak.

Safety: Side effects are uncommon with both vaccines, except mild fever and local reaction. No horizontal transmission has been reported with live vaccine.

Contraindications are none, though dose may be deferred during acute severe febrile illness. Vaccine may be safely given with other childhood vaccines.

Frequently Asked Questions (FAQs)

1. **Whether HAV vaccination is recommended to all children?**

   WHO recommends HAV vaccination in all countries transitioning from high to intermediate endemicity of disease like India, though the cost and logistics preclude its inclusion in NIS. IAP recommends HAV vaccination to all healthy children below 10 yrs of age and in seronegative children beyond 10 years. HAV vaccine is particularly important in high-risk groups.

2. **Which children are at higher risk for HAV infection or severe disease, in whom HAV vaccination is considered as more important?**

   HAV vaccine is particularly important in high risk groups e.g. - a) Chronic liver disease, b) Hepatitis B or C carriers,

c) Immunodeficiency states, d) Transplant recipients, e) Institutionalized children in hostels etc, f) Seronegative adolescents who are leaving home for residential schools, g) Travelers to endemic regions, and h) Household contact with a case (within 10 days).

3. **Why is Pre-vaccination screening recommended above 10 years of age?**

In India, over half of the adolescents and adults are already seropositive due to natural infections in childhood, who are unlikely to benefit from vaccination. As the cost of pre-vaccination antibody screening to identify still susceptible cases is lower than the cost of vaccine, IAP ACVIP recommends it for those above 10 years of age.

4. **Which HAV vaccine is preferable – Inactivated or Live?**

Live vaccine has been shown to be marginally more protective for pre-exposure prophylaxis i.e. ~100% vs 90-95% with Inactivated vaccines. Otherwise, all licensed vaccines have nearly similar efficacy. Live vaccine cannot be used in immunocompromised patients.

5. **Whether a single dose of inactivated HAV may be used, if two doses are not possible?**

While studies have shown higher antibody titers achieved after two doses than the one dose, a single dose is as protective as two doses in immunocompetent persons, apart from being less expensive. Many countries have successfully used single dose schedule in national programs. In fact, considering the disease burden and effectiveness of single dose, IAP recommends inclusion of a single dose HAV in the NIS. However, two-dose schedule is preferred in immunocompromized and high-risk population.

6. **Whether HAV vaccine may be given during pregnancy?**

Yes. Unvaccinated or partially vaccinated pregnant women can be and should be vaccinated for the same indications as non-pregnant women.

7. Can HAV vaccine be given to immunocompromised people?

Yes. Inactivated HAV should be given to all immunocompromised people, specially those on dialysis or having HIV. Live vaccine cannot be used in them.

8. What is the role of HAV vaccine in Post-exposure prophylaxis following exposure?

Single dose vaccine provides effective post-exposure prophylaxis against HAV when given within 2 weeks of exposure and has been used successfully to control outbreaks in many countries. *Post-exposure prophylaxis* is indicated in household contacts above one year of age within 10 days of exposure with a single dose, though it is better to complete the immunization later with second dose (Total 2 doses). Immunoglobulins (IM 0.02–0.06 ml/Kg) may be used in infants or immunocompromized children.

Key points

- **Vaccine:** Inactivated and Live attenuated vaccines, also available in combination with HBV

- **Dose:** *Inactivated: 0.5 ml IM (1 ml> 19 yrs age)*

  Live Attenuated: 0.5 ml SC

- **Immunization Schedule:** Not included in NIS, IAP recommends after 12 mo of age as follows -

  Inactivated: Two doses at 6-18 mo interval (12-23 mo), No Boosters

  Live Attenuated: Single dose (1-15 years), No Boosters

- **Catchup immunization:** Two doses at 0,6 mo (Single dose for live vaccine)

  After Pre-vaccination screening beyond 10 yrs age

  Three doses at 0,1,6 mo for Combination (HAV+HBV)

- **Efficacy:** Inactivated: 90-95%, Live attenuated: 100%

- **Safety:** Side-effects uncommon, except mild fever and local reaction

- **Contraindications:** Immunocompromized states (for Live vaccine only)

References

1. World Health Organization. Hepatitis A Vaccines: Position paper: Weekly Epid. Record 2012;87:261-276.
2. Pemde HK. Hepatitis A vaccines: *In:* IAP Guidebook on Immunization 2018-19 - Advisory Committee on Vaccines and Immunization Practices, Indian Academy of Pediatrics, 3rd Edition, New Delhi, Jaypee Brothers 2020; pp 265-277.
3. Narain NP. Hepatitis A *In:* Vashishtha V et al. FAQs on Vaccines and immunization practices. 2nd Edition. .New Delhi, Jaypee Brothers 2015; pp 173-179.

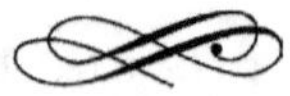

Varicella-zoster virus (VCZ) infection presents either as a primary infection, i.e. *Chickenpox* or as re-activation of earlier latent infection, i.e. H*erpes zoster*.

Epidemiology: VCZ is a neurotropic human herpes virus, present in respiratory secretions or vesicles of a case and transmitted via direct contact or as droplet infection. Infection is highly contagious with secondary attack rate of 80–90% in household contacts and 30–35% in schoolmates. Transplacental fetal infection is possible in pregnant mothers with VCZ infection.

Chickenpox is most common in toddlers and early school children, though no age is immune, including newborns. Disease tends to be more severe in older children/adults and in immunocompromized population. Outbreaks are common during winter and spring season.

Infection generally confers life-long immunity, but virus stays in tissues in a dormant state and reactivation may occur as Herpes-zoster after many years in ~10% cases, specially in immunocompromized states.

Vaccine: Varicella vaccine is a live-attenuated monovalent vaccine, prepared from *Oka strain* of virus, with each dose containing minimum 1000 plaque forming units (PFU). Developed by Takahashi et al., Japan and first licensed in 1984; all currently available varicella vaccines are derived from same strain.

Varicella vaccine is also available in combination with Measles, Mumps and Rubella vaccine as quadrivalent MMRV (Priorix tetra®).

Contents & storage: All varicella vaccines, including MMRV, are supplied as a single-dose lyophilized powder with diluents. To be stored at 2–8°C for 24-36 months and protected from light, vaccine should be used within 30 minutes after reconstitution.

Dosage & administration: Varicella vaccine is given subcutaneously as 0.5 ml/dose.

Immunization Schedule: Minimum age for varicella vaccination is 12 months. While not included in NIS, IAP recommends varicella vaccine to all children without past history of varicella, in the age group of 15 months to 18 years, with *two doses - first dose at or after 15 months of age and second dose preferably after 3-6 months*. However, high-risk children must be given two doses at shorter 4-8 weeks interval.

Catch-up immunization is recommended for all children below 18 years of age without documented history of age-appropriate vaccination or varicella/Herpes zoster disease or laboratory evidence of immunity, with two doses at interval of 3 months (4-8 weeks in high risk children or older adolescents > 13 years). Varicella vaccination is particularly more important in some high-risk children (FAQ 2).

MMR+V or MMRV: Considering higher frequency of adverse events with MMRV in 12-23 months age group, IAP recommends that the first dose of varicella at 15 months should be given as stand-alone varicella vaccine with separate MMR vaccine (MMR+V), while second dose at 5 years may be given as a combination vaccine (MMRV) or separately (MMR+V), as per parent's choice. MMRV is licensed only till 12 years of age.

Efficacy: All varicella vaccines are equally immunogenic and induce both humoral and cellular immunity. Seroprotection rate is higher with two doses (>99%) than the single dose (~86%). Immunogenicity is lower in adolescents and adults than in younger children. Antibody titers drop with time though persistence of protective levels has been reported even after 10 years after single dose. Cell mediated T cell proliferation responses persist in 87–90% of children for up to 5 years.

Protective efficacy is higher against moderate to severe disease (>99%) than the mild disease (70-75%). Varicella vaccine has also been shown to prevent herpes zoster in elderly people with ~ 50% reduction in incidence.

Studies comparing two doses of MMR + V (both vaccines given separately) and MMRV (combination vaccine) have shown adequate seroconversion for all four antigens.

Safety: Side-effects are mild and transient, including local reactions and fever. Adverse events e.g. high fever, rash and febrile seizures more common in children not primed earlier with Measles containing vaccine e.g. those receiving MMRV as first dose than MMR+V separately. Other important side effects include modified varicella like illness, Breakthrough varicella and Herpes zoster.

Modified Varicella like illness (MVLI), seen in < 5% vaccinees, presents as mild papulovesicular eruptions after 1–3 weeks, lasting for few days.

Breakthrough varicella is defined as a clinical disease after 42 days of immunization (d/d MVLI, within 1-3 weeks), usually seen in 1-4% vaccinees within 2–5 years of vaccination. It is more common in children vaccinated <15 months of age or in late childhood, received steroids within 3 months or received varicella vaccine within 28 days of MMR vaccine but not on the same day. Breakthrough disease is usually mild, with <50 skin lesions, predominantly maculopapular rather than vesicular rash, low or no fever, and shorter duration of illness. However, these cases are contagious and may cause outbreaks or severe disease in immunocompromised patients.

Breakthrough varicella represents Inadequate immune response, specially the memory T-cell response, leading to waning of immunity over time. Two doses provide higher geometric mean antibody titers and reduce the risk of breakthrough varicella by 3.3 fold than the single dose. However Vaccine failure after single dose is mainly 'primary' as most cases of breakthrough disease occur within five years of vaccination.

Herpes zoster is known to occur with both, wild and vaccine virus, in vaccinated children though incidence is less than in unvaccinated children. Since the children with post-vaccination breakthrough disease are co-infected with both wild and vaccine strains, they may be at higher risk for herpes zoster in later life.

Safety concerns due to presence of traces of adjuvants and stabilizers e.g. Monosodium glutamate, Gelatin, Trehalose, neomycin and Human albumin, in some varicella vaccines seems to be unfounded.

Contraindications: Being a live vaccine, it should not be given to severely immunocompromized children i.e. - a) HIV with CD4 count less than 15% or 200 cells/mm^3, b) Leukemia till not in remission and off chemotherapy for 3 months and c) Long-term (>14 days) high-dose steroids (>2 mg/kg Prednisolone equivalent) till stopped for 4 weeks. It may be given in cases on low-dose or alternate-day steroids.

Salicylates should be avoided for 6 weeks post-vaccination due to potential risk of Reye syndrome.

Vaccine is contraindicated during pregnancy and when used in adult females, pregnancy should be avoided for 3 months after vaccination.

Frequently Asked Questions (FAQs)

1. **Why is varicella vaccine not yet included in NIS?**

   Varicella vaccine is not recommended for universal immunization in India as the disease is generally mild and vaccine is expensive. Moreover, universal immunization will be beneficial only if high and sustained coverage is possible. Low vaccine coverage (< 80%) might shift the age-epidemiology of the disease towards adults, who often have more severe disease.

2. **Which children require varicella vaccination on priority, if not given routinely?**

   Varicella vaccination is particularly more important in some high-risk children i.e. - a) Chronic lung or heart disease, b) Immunocompromized states including HIV, Malignancy, chemotherapy and steroid therapy, barring some contraindications, discussed later, c) Household contacts of immunocompromized children, d) Institutionalized children attending crèches, day-care centers or orphanages, etc. e) Adolescents who have not had varicella in past and are varicella IgG negative, especially if they are leaving home for a residential school/college.

3. **Why is first dose of varicella recommended at 15 months of age, when the vaccine is licensed for use after 12 months?**

   Risk of breakthrough varicella is lower if vaccine is given

after 15 months of age. However, during outbreaks, the vaccine may be given from 12 months onwards.

4. Why is second dose recommended for regular immunization after 3-6 months, unlike prior recommendation at the age of 4–6 years?

IAP has changed its recommendation regarding second dose after 3-6 months of first dose rather than at 4-6 years of age with following rationale -

- Timing of the second dose would depend on the relative contributions of primary and secondary vaccine failure to the incidence of breakthrough varicella. Primary vaccine failure to seroconvert after first dose favors an early second dose (after 3-6 mo) while secondary vaccine failure due to gradual waning of immunity over time favor a late second dose (at 4-6 years).

- While seroprotective titers after second dose are similar irrespective of the timing of second dose, Geometric mean titers (GMT) and Mean stimulation index (MSI)- a marker of cell mediated immunity, are superior with longer time intervals. Hence, the earlier recommendation favored second dose at 4-6 years of age.

- However, recent studies have shown persistence or even rise of protective antibody titers for 10-20 years after vaccination due to natural boosting. Since most cases of breakthrough varicella occur within 4-5 years of first dose, primary vaccine failure seems to be more important than secondary vaccine failure in etiology and hence, the recommendations have been revised in favor of second dose after 3-6 months of first dose.

5. Which vaccine brand is better for varicella immunization considering wide differences in the reported immunogenicity of vaccines?

All currently available vaccines are equally effective and safe, derived from same strain and differ only in their viral content and adjuvants. Reported differences in the immunogenicity are largely due to use of different correlates of seroprotection e.g. a correlate of gp-ELISA >5 units/ml was achieved by 86% after single dose, while studies using fluorescent antibody to membrane antigen (FAMA) titers of >1:4 after 16 weeks as the cut-off found that only 76% vaccinees achieved it.

6. **Whether MMRV can be used instead of MMR and Varicella vaccines given separately?**

Two doses of MMR + V (separately) and MMRV (combination vaccine) have shown adequate and comparable seroconversion for all four antigens with both options. However, adverse events e.g. high fever, rash and febrile seizures are more common with MMRV in children below 2 years. Hence, IAP recommends that the first dose at 15 months should be given separately as MMR+V while second dose at 5 years may be as per parent's choice - MMRV or MMR+V.

7. **Whether a 13 year old girl, unimmunized with MMR earlier may be given MMRV to cover four viral infections?**

MMRV is licensed only till 12 years of age and cannot be used for catch-up immunization of adolescents.

8. **Whether varicella vaccine can cause Herpes zoster?**

Herpes Zoster is known to occur with both – wild and vaccine virus, in varicella vaccinated children though incidence is less than in unvaccinated children. Since the children with post-vaccination breakthrough disease are co-infected with both wild and vaccine strains, they may be at higher risk for herpes zoster in later life.

9. **Whether Varicella vaccine can be used for prevention of Herpes zoster?**

A recent systematic review has suggested the efficacy of vaccination to prevent herpes zoster in elderly people, demonstrating almost 50% reduction in incidence. However, longer follow-up studies are needed for confirmation due to very long latent period between primary infection and Herpes Zoster.

A specific Herpes zoster vaccine, containing same VZV Oka strain but with much higher antigenic load (minimum 19400 PFU) is licensed in some countries for use in persons > 50 years, given as single dose of 0.65 ml subcutaneously.

10. **Whether varicella vaccine can be used for post-exposure prophylaxis?**

Varicella vaccine within 5 days of exposure has been shown to have more than 80% efficacy against moderate to severe disease. However, it is contraindicated in Immunocompromized states and pregnancy.

11. **What are the indication for Post-exposure prophylaxis in contacts?**

Post-exposure prophylaxis is indicated in *susceptible* (unvaccinated or without laboratory evidence of prior disease) and *exposed* (> 1 hour contact in same room with a case of varicella in infectivity period or Herpes Zoster) persons with following high-risk attributes – a) immunocompromised states*, b) Pregnancy; c) newborns of mothers who develop varicella within 5 days before or 2 days after the delivery, d) All preterm newborns less than 28 weeks/1000 gm, exposed in neonatal period, and e) Preterm newborns > 28 weeks with mothers negative for anti-varicella IgG.

* Note: Marrow transplant recipients are considered susceptible even if they had disease or received vaccinations prior to transplant. Immunocompromised children who have received IVIG 400 mg/kg is past 3 weeks are considered as protected.

> **Key points**
>
> - **Vaccine:** Live attenuated (Oka strain), also available as Combination vaccine (MMRV)
>
> - **Formulation:** Single-dose, Lyophilized 0.5 ml / dose, Subcutaneously
>
> - **Immunization Schedule:** Not in NIS, IAP recommends -
>
>   *Regular:* Two doses at/after 15 months with 3-6 months interval
>
>   *High-risk:* Two doses at 4-8 weeks interval
>
> - **Catch-up Immunization:** Upto 18 years,
>
>   *Children till 13 years age*: Two doses at 3 mo interval
>
>   *High-risk children or adolescents > 13 years*: Two doses at 4-8 week interval
>
> - **Efficacy:** > 99% for moderate/severe disease, 70-90% for mild disease
>
> - **Safety:** Side-effects uncommon, except mild fever and local reaction.
>
>   Rarely, MVLI, Break-through varicella, H. zoster
>
> - **Contraindication:** Immunocompromized states, Pregnancy, salicylate therapy

12. What are the options for Post-exposure prophylaxis in contacts?

Best option for the Post-exposure prophylaxis in susceptible and exposed contacts is Passive prophylaxis with Varicella zoster immunoglobulin (VZIG), given within 10 days of exposure.

Currently available VZIG (Varitect® 25 IU/ml) and is given IV as 0.2-1ml/ kg diluted in normal saline over 1 hour. Efficacy is highest (~100%) against death in exposed newborns and duration of protection lasts for 3 weeks. Side effects include allergic reactions and anaphylaxis. As VZIG prolongs the incubation period, all VZIG recipients should be monitored for at least 28 weeks for disease manifestations.

Other alternatives for Post exposure prophylaxis include –

a) PO Acyclovir from 7th to 21st day of exposure as

80 mg/kg/day (or PO 200 mg QID <2 years, 400 mg QID for 2-6 years or 800 mg QID above 6 years of age).

b) Varicella vaccine (see FAQ 10).

c) IV immunoglobulin 200 mg/kg Single dose within 10 days, though protective efficacy is not known.

References

1. World Health Organization. Varicella and Herpes zoster vaccines: Position paper: Weekly Epid. Record 2014;89: 265-288.

2. Shah AK. Varicella Vaccines: *In:* IAP Guidebook on Immunization 2018-19 - Advisory Committee on Vaccines and Immunization Practices, Indian Academy of Pediatrics, 3rd Edition, New Delhi, Jaypee Brothers 2020; pp 246-264.

3. Yewle V et al Varicella *In:* Vashishtha V et al. FAQs on Vaccines and immunization practices. 2nd Edition. New Delhi, Jaypee Brothers 2015; pp 180-194.

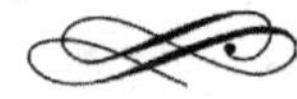

Influenza Vaccines

Influenza is a highly contagious viral illness of respiratory tract with seasonal outbreaks *(seasonal influenza)* as well as intermittent pandemics *(pandemic influenza)*.

Seasonal influenza is common in winter season and outbreaks tend to subside after 4–6 weeks with low morbidity and mortality. Globally, It is estimated to affect 5-10% of population annually, specially children, though less than 1-2% of them have life-threatening lower respiratory disease.

Pandemic influenza involves a particularly contagious strain of virus that spread rapidly to create large-scale pandemics.Past century has witnessed four global influenza pandemics, including the current H1N1 pandemic (Swine flu) since 2009. Earlier pandemics began in 1918 due to H1N1 (Spanish flu), 1957 due to H2N2 (Asian flu) and 1968 due to H3N2 (HongKong flu), with 1918 pandemic being most severe leading to estimated 20–40 million deaths.

Epidemiology: Influenza is a large RNA virus with three major serotypes affecting humans – A, B, and C. While all pandemics have been caused only by serotype A, seasonal outbreaks are usually due to A and B serotypes. Type C virus is responsible for rare, sporadic and mild upper respiratory tract infections.

Serotype A is further classified on the basis of two surface proteins – Hemagglutinin (HA) and Neuraminidase (NA) and strains are named on the basis of the combination of HA and NA proteins, e.g. H1N1, H2N2, H3N2, etc. Nomenclature of influenza virus includes virus serotype, geographic origin, strain no, year of isolation and virus subtype in order e.g. A/California/7/2009/H1N1.

Epidemiology of influenza is interesting as prevalent strains are known to change every year following minor antigenic changes due to point mutations (antigenic drift), and less frequently following major antigenic changes due to reassortment of viral gene segments with emergence of novel subtype (Antigenic shift). This novel subtype, then, tends to replace existing seasonal viruses leading to pandemics, and subsequently, after development of partial herd immunity, continues to circulate as the new seasonal virus. Thereafter it would exhibit antigenic drift; thus more than one drifted variant may co-circulate at the same time. Antigenic shifts occur only in serotype A, while antigenic drifts occur in both serotype A & B.

Latest global pandemic, caused by novel influenza strain (H1N1), was originated in USA in 2009 and initially affected pigs (Swine flu). India was affected soon after with first case in May 2009. Now, this pandemic has gradually weakened with development of herd immunity and most cases occur as seasonal outbreaks or endemic disease due to H1N1, H3N2 and serotype B infections.

In India, Seasonal influenza peaks during winter in north India (Northern global hemisphere pattern) and during monsoons or post-monsoon season in other parts of country (Southern global hemisphere pattern).

Vaccine: Influenza vaccines are Trivalent or Quadrivalent. All trivalent vaccines contain two serotype A and one serotype B seasonal strains while quadrivalent vaccines include one additional serotype B strain i.e. two strains each of serotype A and B. WHO recommends two different set of vaccine strains every year depending on prevalent strains in previous season, one for Northern hemisphere in the month of February and another for southern hemisphere countries in September.

For the year 2020-21 season, WHO has recommended following strains for trivalent northern hemisphere vaccines - *A/Victoria/2570/2019 (H1N1)pdm09-like virus; A/Cambodia/ e0826360/2020 (H3N2)-like virus; B/Washington/02/2019 (B/Victoria lineage)-like virus* and following strains for southern hemispehere - A/Victoria/2570/2019 (H1N1) pdm09-like virus; A/Hong Kong/2671/2019 (H3N2)-like virus; and B/Washington/02/2019 (B/Victoria lineage)-like virus; Quadrivalent vaccines for this season also include one B/ Phuket/3073/2013-like virus (B/Yamagata lineage), for both hemispheres. All current influenza vaccines include Pandemic 2009 H1N1 strain and no separate vaccine is required.

Although entire India geographically lies in northern hemisphere, southern hemisphere vaccines are considered as more appropriate in this country, especially for south India.

Biologically, two types of influenza vaccines are available globally - (a) Inactivated and (b) live attenuated., Live attenuated influenza vaccines are presently not available in India.

19.1: INACTIVATED INFLUENZA VACCINES (IIV)

IIV are usually split-virion trivalent or quadrivalent vaccines (or subunit surface-antigen formulations), produced from highly purified and inactivated virus grown on embryonated hen eggs. Quadrivalent vaccines *(Fluquadri®, Vaxiflu-4®, Fluarix-Tetra®, Influvac-Tetra®)* are preferred over trivalent vaccines.

Contents and Storage: IIVs contain 7.5 or 15 µg Hemagglutin of each component strain, supplied as 0.25 or 0.5 ml single-dose vials or prefilled syringes, to be stored on 2–8°C.

Dosage & Administration: To be given Intramuscularly or deep subcutaneously, most manufacturers recommend lower doses of IIV (0.25 ml) below 3 years of age as compared to 0.5 ml in older children and adults due to higher reactogenicity and risk of febrile seizures in younger children.

However, recent studies have shown comparable reactogenicity of new generation split-virion vaccines in younger children with advantage of better immunogenicity against Non-H1N1 strains with higher dose. Hence, currently IAP recommends *uniform dose of 0.5 ml to all children* above 6 months of age, if approved by licensing authorities and recommended by manufacturers.

Immunization Schedule: Influenza vaccine is not included in NIS. IAP recommends Influenza vaccination to all children from 6 months to 5 years of age, and in high-risk children beyond this age vulnerable for severe disease and death. High-risk children include those with –

- Chronic cardiac, pulmonary (excluding asthma), hematologic, renal (including Nephrotic syndrome) and liver disease and Diabetes mellitus;

- Congenital or acquired immunodeficiency, including HIV infection; and

- Long-term salicylates therapy.

For IIVs, minimum age of vaccination is 6 months and previously unvaccinated children below 9 years of age are recommended two doses at 4-week interval in the first year, followed by single dose annually. In children aged 9 years or above, adolescents or adults, only single dose is recommended even if not vaccinated earlier.

All influenza vaccines, IIV or LAIV, have to be repeated annually, preferably just before the onset of peak influenza season, referred earlier.

Efficacy: Humoral response to Influenza vaccines is strain-specific and hence, it is important that this annual vaccine should incorporate the strains expected to be prevalent and recommended for the current year.

Protective efficacy depends on the composition of the vaccine, diagnostic case-definition (clinical Influneza-like illness *vs* laboratory confirmed), previous antigenic exposure (vaccination) and underlying high-risk disease. Post-vaccination, anti-HA antibody titers peak after 2-4 weeks (earlier in previously vaccinated individuals) and fall by ≥50% after 6 months, before stabilizing for next 2-3 years.

Reported protective efficacy of IIVs is ~59% for confirmed influenza and ~36% for influenza-like-illnesses, lasting for at least 6-8 months. Quadrivalent IIVs, though not extensively studied so far, are at least as effective as trivalent IIVs, with added advantage of extra strain.

Side-effects: IIVs are generally safe except for local reactions and transient systemic reactions e.g. fever, malaise and myalgia in some cases, more common after re-vaccinations. There have been reports of marginal but unproven higher incidence of febrile seizures and Guillain barre syndrome (GBS) in some reports. IIVs do not contain thiomersal.

Contraindications: IIVs should be avoided in cases of egg allergy or past history of GBS, unless they are at high-risk for Influenza-related complications. IIVs should also be avoided during acute febrile illnesses.

19.2: LIVE ATTENUATED INFLUENZA VACCINE (LAIV)

LAIV, though manufactured in India (Nasovac-S®) and available globally, is currently not available in India. It is a freeze-dried vaccine, administered as intranasal spray of 0.25 ml in each nostril and is given as single dose annually irrespective of the age. LAIV is contraindicated in high-risk and immunocompromized children or during pregnancy and cannot be used in young children < 2 years. LAIVs, which replicate in nasophayrnx to induce protective immunity, are reported to have better protective efficacy than IIVs (~82% for confirmed influenza and 33% for influenza-like-illnesses). Safety profile is also comparable except local nasal irritation/ stuffiness and flu-like illness.

Frequently Asked Questions (FAQs)

1. **Why is influenza vaccine not included in NIS?**

   Influenza vaccine is not yet included in national program due to lack of sufficient local data on morbidity and mortality. Logistic issues i.e. need for annual re-vaccinations and suitability of a single vaccine for whole country with significant seasonal variations in influenza epidemiology also preclude inclusion of Influenza vaccination in NIS.

2. **Then, who should be offered the Influenza vaccine?**

   IAP recommends influenza vaccination universally to all children till 5 years (6 months of age onwards) and in high-risk children (discussed earlier, Sec 19.1) beyond this age due to vulnerability for severe disease and death.

Other high-risk categories include elderly persons > 65 years, Pregnant women, institutionalized population (e.g. old-age and disabled home dwellers) and occupationally exposed people e.g. Health care workers.

3. **Why does IAP recommends routine influenza vaccination to all Under-five children?**

Influenza accounts for 5-10% of all acute respiratory infections, with incidence as well as severity being higher in younger children and in developing countries. In limited Indian data, incidence of Influenza-associated acute respiratory infections and acute lower respiratory infections during infancy is estimated to be ~180 and 33 per 1000 infants per year respectively.

In view of significant morbidity and higher mortality in younger children, paucity of facilities for laboratory diagnosis, high transmission rate, substantial socioeconomic burden, limitations of oseltamivir and availability of moderately efficacious vaccine, IAP recommends Influenza vaccine routinely in all children below the age of 5 years.

4. **Why does Influenza vaccine has to be given annually?**

Prevalent virus strains change every year due to minor antigenic changes following point mutations (*antigenic drift*), and less frequently due to major antigenic changes with emergence of novel subtype (*Antigenic shift*). Vaccines largely elicit a strain-specific humoral response with none or lesser efficacy against antigenically changed viruses. Hence, the given vaccine should incorporate the current strain prevalent during that time.

To ensure optimal vaccine efficacy against prevailing strains in different geographical regions, antigenic composition of vaccines is revised twice a year by the WHO - one for the northern hemisphere countries (in February) and another for southern hemisphere countries (in September). Manufacturers make these vaccines available within 6 months of the revision.

5. **Which influenza vaccine – with Northern or Southern composition, should be used in India?**

Although India is geographically in northern hemisphere, it is a vast country with different seasonal patterns of influenza in different states - winters in north India and rainy season in other parts of country. Hence, uniform recommendation for whole country is not justifiable and India needs a staggered approach for Influenza vaccination timing.

WHO classifies India under the "South Asia" transmission zone of influenza circulation with peaks during rainy season and southern hemisphere vaccines are considered as more appropriate. Composition for southern vaccine is released in September and vaccines are available by next March-April for use in upcoming season, which is the best time to vaccinate to prevent monsoon outbreaks.

However, some southern Indian states with late monsoon rains (September - December) also have influenza peaks in winters and might benefit from Northern hemisphere vaccines.

6. **So, What is best time to offer Influenza Vaccine to prevent seasonal influenza?**

Influenza vaccine should be offered about 2 weeks before the onset of season in geographic location – Pre-Winter in North India and Pre-Monsoons in rest of the India.

7. **Which Influenza vaccine is better – Live or inactivated and Quadrivalent or trivalent?**

LAIV is not available in India. Further, despite better protective efficacy against laboratory confirmed

Influenza (82% vs 59% with IIVs), it cannot be used in Immunocompromized children as well as during pregnancy.

All IIVs are equally effective, though quadrivalent vaccines offer added benefit against extra strain.

8. **Whether Influenza vaccine can be given during pregnancy?**

Yes. IIVs can be used at any stage of pregnancy. In fact, WHO recommends that Pregnant women should get highest priority for influenza immunization due to higher risk of severe disease and death as well as complications in offsprings e.g. stillbirth, neonatal death, preterm delivery, and low birth weight. Vaccine in pregnancy also protects their young infants from severe disease. However, LAIV is contraindicated during pregnancy.

Key points

- **Vaccine:** Inactivated trivalent or Quadrivalent vaccines (Live attenuated vaccine not available in India)

- **Dose:** IM/SC 0.5 ml/dose (0.25 ml below 3 year, if recommended by the manufacturers)

- **Schedule:** Not in NIS. IAP recommends to all children 6 mo - 5 years, as –

    Two dose at 0, 4 weeks in first year, than

    Single dose annually before peak season.

- **Catch-up immunization:** (Upto 5 years only, except in high-risk cases*)

    < 9 years: Two dose at 0,4 weeks than single dose annually.

    > 9 years: Single dose annually before peak season.

- **Protective efficacy:** ~59% (36% for influenza-like-illnesses) for 6-8 months.

- **Side-effects:** Local reaction, Febrile seizures, Guillaine Barre syndrome,

- **Contraindications:** Egg allergy, H/o GBS, defer during acute febrile illness

---

*see text

References

1. Pemde HK et al. Influenza Vaccines *In:* IAP Guidebook on Immunization 2018-19 - Advisory Committee on Vaccines and Immunization Practices, Indian Academy of Pediatrics, 3rd Edition, New Delhi, Jaypee Brothers 2020; pp 315-332.

2. Sharma S. Influenza *In:* Vashishtha V et al. FAQs on Vaccines and immunization practices. 2nd Edition. New Delhi, Jaypee Brothers 2015; pp 288-295.

3. Saha S et al. Divergent seasonal patterns of influenza types A and B across latitude gradient in Tropical Asia. Influenza Other Respir Viruses 2016;10(3);176-84.

4. World Health Organization Seasonal influenza (inactivated) vaccines: Position paper: Weekly Epid. Record 2012;87:461-476.

5. Vashistha VM. Influenza Vaccination in India: Position Paper of Indian Academy of Pediatrics. Indian Pediatrics, 2013;50: 867-874.

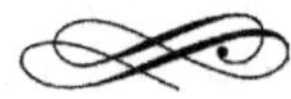

Human Papillomavirus Vaccines

Human papillomavirus (HPV) is the commonest sexually transmitted infection though usually benign and self-limiting. However, persistent infection with some genotypes may lead to development of genital warts or cervical, ano-genital and oropharyngeal cancers after long lag period of 15-20 years. Of these, Cervical cancer, the most dreaded consequence, is the second commonest cancer in Indian women.

Epidemiology: HPV is a DNA virus with over 100 genotypes, of which at least 13 are known to be oncogenic. High-risk HPV type 16 & 18 cause ~70% of invasive cervical cancer while low-risk HPV type 6 & 11 are responsible for ~90% cases of genital warts or recurrent respiratory papillomatosis. In India, over 97% cases of cervical cancers have demonstrated presence of high-risk HPV genotypes, predominantly type 16 in 65% cases, followed by type 18, 45, 33, 35 and others. HPV-16 and HPV-45 are more prevalent in North India while HPV-35 is commoner in South India.

Natural HPV infections are superficial, limited to intraepithelial basement layers of the mucosa and hence, do not induce vigorous immune response. While ~50% of infected women develop detectable antibodies, these are non-neutralizing and not necessarily protective.

HPV genome is a capsid shell comprising major (L1) and minor (L2) structural proteins. Antibodies against L1 viral protein are usually neutralizing and type-specific. All HPV vaccines are recombinant vaccines containing a mixture of the L1 proteins of various vaccine serotypes.

Vaccine: Currently, two HPV vaccines are available in India - a *bivalent* vaccine (HPV2) containing serotypes 16 & 18 and a *quadrivalent* vaccine (HPV4) containing two more serotypes 6 & 11, in addition to 16 & 18. A nine-valent vaccine with further additional serotypes 31, 33, 45, 52, and 58 (Gardasil-9®) will also be available shortly in India.

Contents and storage: Both HPV2 and HPV4 are single dose 0.5 ml suspension, to be stored at 2–8°C.

Dosage & administration: All HPV vaccines are to be given as 0.5 ml/dose intramuscularly in deltoid region.

Immunization Schedule: Not included in NIS, HPV vaccines in India are licensed for use only in females from 9 to 26 years of age, given as three doses at 0, 1, 6 months (for HPV2) or 0, 2, 6 months (for HPV4).

However, IAP recommends two-dose schedule at 0, 6 months for younger girls aged 9-14 years, which is equally immunogenic provided the dose-interval is *not less than* 5 months. Else, a third dose must be given after 5 months of first dose or 12 weeks of second dose. For older girls ≥15 years or in immunocompromised states, only three-dose schedule is recommended.

Vaccination should be initiated as early as possible, preferably at 9 years of age as HPV vaccines do not protect against the serotype with which the infection has already occurred before vaccination. Immune response is also higher in pre-adolescent vaccinees *versus* in adolescents and young adults. Catch-up vaccination is permitted till 45 years of age.

Efficacy: Mechanisms of protection is not fully defined but seem to involve both cellular immunity and neutralizing IgG antibodies. Correlates of protection are not well established. Vaccines do not impact the outcome of HPV-16/18 infections present at the time of vaccination. For vaccine virus genotypes not previously infected, both vaccines are equally immunogenic i.e. ~90%. In cases already infected with one vaccine genotype, vaccines have been found to be effective against other constituent genotypes. Protective IgG titers are reported to persist in >90% cases after 8-9 years.

Protective efficacy against cervical cancer is difficult to assess due to long lag period between the HPV infection and invasive disease. Currently, protective efficacy against cervical intraepithelial neoplasia (CIN 2/3) and adenocarcinoma *in situ* caused by vaccine strains has been accepted as the end-point of efficacy trials. Using these parameters, both vaccines have been found to be equally effective against cervical cancer and pre-cancerous lesions.

Protective efficacy of HPV2 vaccine is >90% in women without evidence of prior or current HPV 16/18 infection, though relatively lower (~70-80%) in cases with previous infections. HPV4 vaccine has marginally higher >98% protective efficacy against constituent-genotype related precancerous conditions, lasting for over five years.

HPV4 vaccine also protects against anogenital warts due to presence of low-risk genotypes 6 and 11, and has shown an efficacy of >65% against external genital warts in males. Interestingly, HPV2 vaccine, which does not contain these genotypes, has also been found to reduce the incidence of external genital warts by 30-50%, suggesting some cross-protection against non-constituent genotype infections.

Safety: Both vaccines are safe, except local pain and swelling for 24-48 hours. Fever may occur in <10% cases. Syncope following vaccination is known specially in adolescents and it is advisable to observe vaccinees for 15-30 minutes after vaccination.

Contraindications: Both vaccines are contraindicated in those with history of hypersensitivity to any component or previous dose and should be avoided in pregnancy. Vaccines may be given to immunocompromised patients though immunogenicity may not be optimal.

Frequently Asked Questions (FAQs)

1. **Whether HPV is an anti-cancer vaccine?**

   HPV vaccine is not an anti-cancer vaccine in true sense but prevents high-risk HPV infections, associated with ~70% of invasive cervical cancer. In India, over 97% cases of cervical cancers have demonstrated presence of high-risk HPV genotypes. Accordingly, IAP suggests promotion of these vaccines as against cervical cancer rather than against sexually transmitted infections.

2. **Whether HPV vaccine should be included in the National immunization program?**

   WHO recommends introduction of HPV vaccine in NIS of the countries with high burden of cervical cancer like India, though cost and logistics preclude it at present. IAP has not yet recommended inclusion of these vaccines in NIS but should be offered to all females, preferably during pre-sexual activity age.

3. **Which vaccine is preferable – HPV2 or HPV4?**

   Both vaccines are equally effective but HPV4 also offers protection against genital warts due to inclusion of low-risk genotypes 6 and 11. However, HPV2 (without these genotypes) has also been found to reduce the incidence of external genital warts by 30-50%, suggesting some cross-protection against non-constituent genotype infections.

4. **Considering the wide age-group recommendations for HPV vaccines, what should be the ideal age for HPV vaccinations?**

   HPV vaccines are licensed for use from 9-26 years

of age with catch-up immunization permitted till 45 years. However, these vaccines do not protect against the serotypes with which the infection has already occurred before vaccination. As the risk of HPV infections increases progressively with onset of reproductive age, HPV vaccination should be initiated as early as possible, preferably by 10-12 years.

5. **A 16 year old girl received first dose of HPV at the age of 12 years but did not turn up for second dose till now. How many doses must be given to her now?**

    IAP recommends that two doses of HPV vaccine (0,6 mo) are equally immunogenic in girls below 15 years. Since the girl has received first dose before 15 years of age, she is expected to have enough immunogenic stimulation and development of memory cells for good secondary response and now a single dose (total two doses) must be given to her. *Three doses are essential if the first dose was given after 15 years of age.*

6. **A 12 year old girl has received two doses of HPV vaccine at 3 months interval . Is it OK?**

    IAP recommends that two doses are enough in girls below 15 years *provided the time-interval between them is not less than 5 months.* Since in this case dose-interval was only 3 months, a third dose must be given after 5 months of first dose or 12 weeks of second dose. For older girls $\geq$15 years or in immunocompromised states, only three-dose schedule is recommended.

7. **Whether HPV immunized girls also need periodic screening for cervical cancer?**

    HPV vaccines are not 100% protective against cervical cancer and do not protect against an already infected high-risk genotype before vaccination. Hence, HPV vaccination is not a replacement for periodic screening for cervical cancer, which should continue.

8. Whether HPV vaccine is needed in Boys?

HPV4 may also be used in boys with similar schedule to prevent genital warts and anogenital cancers and has been licensed for the same in some countries but not yet in India (for males).

Key points

- **Vaccine:** Recombinant – Bivalent HPV2 (16, 18) or Quadrivalent HPV4 (6, 11, 16, 18).
- **Formulation:** Single-dose 0.5. ml IM
- **Immunization Schedule:** Not in NIS, IAP recommends in 9–26 years age-group as follows -
    - 9–15 years : Two doses at 0, 6 months
    - > 15 years: Three doses at 0, 1, 6 mo (0, 2, 6 mo for HPV4)
- **Catch-up Immunization:** Upto 45 years
- **Efficacy** against HPV infection: ~90% for vaccine genotypes
    - Precancerous conditions: 75% (HPV2) – 98% (HPV4)
    - Anogenital warts: 65% (HPV4), 30–50% with HPV2
- **Safety:** Side-effects uncommon, except mild fever and local reaction.
- **Contraindications** none, except Pregnancy

References

1. World Health Organization. Human Paillomavius vaccines: Position paper.: Weekly Epid. Record 2017;92:241-268.
2. Pemde HK. Huma Papilloma virus vaccines: *In:* IAP Guidebook on Immunization 2018-19 - Advisory Committee on Vaccines and Immunization Practices, Indian Academy of Pediatrics, 3rd Edition, New Delhi, Jaypee Brothers 2020; pp 302-314
3. Choudhury J. Human Paillomavirus In: Vashishtha V et al. FAQs on Vaccines and immunization practices. 2nd Edition. New Delhi, Jaypee Brothers 2015; pp 277-287.

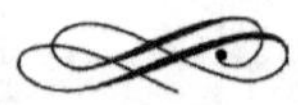

Section

IV

Vaccines for Selective Use

Meningococcal Vaccines

Meningococcal infections in India usually occur in small outbreaks, though disease is endemic in many developed countries. Clinical spectrum ranges from asymptomatic colonization to severe meningitis or systemic meningococcemia with shock. Chronic meningococcemia or non-neurological focal disease is rare in childhood. Meningococci contribute to only 1-2% cases of meningitis in under-five Indian children, though true incidence might be higher due to frequent under-diagnosis. Meningococcal meningitis carries high case-fatality rates (5–15%) or residual neurological sequelae in ~20%.

Epidemiology: *Neisseria meningitides* is a gram-negative bacteria with 13 known serotypes, of which five - A, B, C, Y and W-135 are responsible for ~90% cases. Group A infections are more common in India, while group B, C and Y disease dominate in developed countries.

Humans are only known natural reservoir, with organisms present as commensal in upper respiratory tract of ~ 10% population at any given time. However, this colonization rate may reach as high as 100% during outbreaks.

Infection is highly contagious, transmitted as droplet infection. Disease is most common in preschool children as infants below three months are usually protected by maternal antibodies and older children are relatively protected by antibodies acquired during previous colonization/infection. However, all age groups, including adults, may be affected during outbreaks, which are usually seen in dry winter months. Children with complement-deficiency states, e.g.

nephrotic syndrome, hepatic failure and autoimmune disorders, are more susceptible for meningococcal infections. **Vaccines:** Two types of meningococcal vaccines are available - *Polysaccharide* vaccines (MPSV) and *Conjugate* vaccines (MCV). Of these, MPSV are T-cell independent vaccines, which do not induce immunological memory and are poorly immunogenic in children below 2 years of age.

21.1: MENINGOCOCCAL POLYSACCHARIDE VACCINES (MPSV)

MPSV are generally quadrivalent vaccines containing four serotypes -A,C,W-135,Y (Mencivax®, Quadrimeningo®), though bivalent (A+C) or trivalent vaccines (A+C+W135) are also available.

Contents & storage: Quadrivalent (MPSV4) vaccines contain 50 µg each of the individual polysaccharides of four serotypes (A,C,W-135,Y) in lyophilized form, to be reconstituted with 0.5 ml sterile water. It should be stored at 2 to 8°C.

Dosage & administration: All MPSVs are given as 0.5 ml/dose subcutaneously over thigh or deltoid region.

Immunization schedule: Meningococcal vaccination is not recommended for healthy children, indicated *only* in high-risk population (FAQ 2), preferably using a conjugate vaccine, discussed later. MPSV may be used *if MCV is not feasible*, in – a) High-risk children above two years of age, as a single dose, repeated every 3-5 years, b) during outbreaks or in close-contacts as a single dose above 2 years of age and two doses 3 months apart from 3-24 months of age

Efficacy: Antibody response is serotype-specific with seroconversion rate of >90% in children 2-5 years and ~100%

in older ones, after 10-14 days of vaccination. Vaccine is poorly immunogenic in younger children and is not recommended below 2 years of age except during outbreaks.

Protective efficacy against the clinical disease is >85% in children above 5 years and adults. Protective value in 2-5 years age group is not well established but seems to appropriate at least for the commonest serotype A .

MPSV are T-cell independent vaccines which do not induce immunological memory and antibody titers wane substantially after 2-3 years. Hence, revaccination is required every 3-5 years in high-risk children. Multiple doses are known to cause immunologic hyporesponsiveness, though the impact on clinical efficacy is uncertain.

Safety: MPSV4 is safe though fever and local reactions are common, as also transient irritability, drowsiness, myalgia and gastrointestinal upset in some cases. Local axillary lymphadenopathy is also common.

Contraindications are none except the hypersensitivity to previous dose or vaccine constituents.

21.2: MENINGOCOCCAL CONJUGATE VACCINES (MCV)

MCVs are generally quadrivalent vaccines containing A, C, W135, Y serotypes (menectra®, Menveo®) or monovalent for A serotype (MenAfriVac®). Monovalent vaccine is not available in India, though licensed here and widely used in African countries.

Contents & Storage: Quadrivalent vaccines (MCV4) contains purified polysachharides of four serotypes - A, C, W-135,Y in variable strengths conjugated with diphtheria toxin as carrier protein. Monovalent vaccine (MCV1) contains purified polysachharide of serotype A only, conjugated with tetanus toxoid as carrier protein. All MCVs should be stored at 2 to 8°C.

Dose & administration: All MCVs are given as 0.5 ml Intramuscularly over deltoid region.

Immunization schedule: MCV4 is licensed in India only for persons aged 2–55 years as a single dose, though Menactra® may be used in children aged 9-23 months with two doses at 3 months interval during outbreaks or contact. Meningococcal vaccination is recommended only in select population as follows :

a) In high-risk cases (FAQ2) with two doses at least 8 weeks apart followed by a booster dose every 5 years (First booster after 3 years, if primary series was given before 7 years);

b) During outbreaks, as a single dose from 3 months of age onwards*.

c) In close contacts aged above 3 months, as a single dose within 72 hours of exposure*;

d) Laboratory or Health care workers at risk of exposure, as a single dose, with booster every five years, if exposure is ongoing;

e) International travelers to endemic countries,(FAQ4) as a single dose.

* Note: If MCV is not available, two doses of MPSV three months apart may be used in children aged 3 mo – 2 years. IAP suggests that monovalent MCV may be used for mass vaccination during outbreaks for individuals aged 1–29 years.

Efficacy: MCV4 is highly immunogenic with seroprotective titers in 96-100% after 30 days and persisting for 3-5 years in more than 85% cases.

Seroconversion rate and antibody titers achieved by MCV1 against serotype A are higher and more persistent though declines gradually and only about 50% vaccinees continue to have protective titers after 5 years. Considering that >90% of Indian cases are due to serotype A, IAP recommends availability of this vaccine in India.

Safety: Side-effects are usually minor e.g. local reactions and transient fever. Guillain-Barré Syndrome (GBS) has been reported in some adolescents following MCV4 immunization, though risk is unproven.

Contraindications are none though persons with past history of GBS should avoid it, unless at high-risk for meningococcal disease.

Frequently Asked Questions (FAQs)

1. **What are the indications for meningococcal vaccination?**

    Meningococcal vaccination is not routinely recommended for healthy children, advised only in - a) High-risk children, b) At-risk Health care or Laboratory workers, c) during outbreaks or in close contacts, and d) International travelers to endemic countries.

2. **Which high-risk children need meningococcal vaccination?**

    High-risk children requiring Meningococcal vaccination include those with - a) complement-deficiency states, e.g. nephrotic syndrome, hepatic failure and autoimmune disorders, b) Immunodeficiency states e.g. HIV, and c) Functional or anatomic asplenia/hyposplenia, including sickle cell disease and post-splenectomy.

3. **Which vaccine is preferable in high-risk children – MPSV or MCV?**

    MCV is always preferred over MPSV due to better

immunogenicity specially in those below two years of age and potential for herd protection. Monovalent MCV1 can also be used in India as >90% of Indian cases are due to serotype A, though not available here at present.

4. **What are the meningococcal vaccination requirements for International travelers?**

Meningococcal vaccination requirements vary with country of travel, as follows –

- *Students going for study abroad*, specially USA, generally need a single dose of MCV4 in preceding 5 years with documentation. In USA, MCV4 is a part of routine immunization with single dose MCV4 at 11–12 years followed by a booster at 16 years.

- Haj pilgrims beyond 2 years of age also need a single dose, preferably using MCV4 (not MCV1), within preceding 3 years before the travel.

- Travelers to African countries with meningitis belt need a Single dose of MCV4 or MCV1 with a booster, if last dose was received more than 5 years ago.

5. **What are the meningococcal vaccination requirements during outbreaks?**

Meningococcal outbreak is defined as an attack rate of more than 10 cases/Lac population (or > 3 cases in a given locality within 3 months). Mass vaccination is recommended during such outbreaks using single dose of MCV above three months of age, including in pregnant mothers. MPSV with two doses three months apart can be used, if MCV is not available. Mass vaccination may be stopped if no new case develops for 2 months as secondary cases are unlikely after 10-14 days of contact.

6. **Whether meningococcal vaccination can be used in all outbreaks?**

Currently available Meningococcal vaccines do not

contain serotype B and hence not useful for outbreaks due to serotype B.

7. *What is the post-exposure prophylaxis for close contacts of a meningococcal case?*

All close-contacts of meningococcal case, house-hold or health-worker, should receive chemoprophylaxis with Rifampicin (PO 10 mg/kg BD for 2 days) *or* a single dose of ciprofloxacin or ceftriaxone. As penicillin does not eradicate nasopharyngeal carriage, even index case should receive chemoprophylaxis before discharge, if treated with penicillin.

A single dose of MCV4 or MPSV (if MCV is not available) is also indicated in close household contacts along with chemoprophylaxis.

8. **When should a case planned for splenectomy to receive Meningococal vaccine?**

A prospective splenectomy case should receive a single dose of MCV or MPSV at least two weeks before surgery, followed by a second dose of MCV after 3 months (may be given after surgery) to complete high-risk immunization and boosters every 3-5 years.

9. **Whether PCV and MCV can be given together in a case planned for Splenectomy?**

Some studies have observed interference with PCV13 immune responses, when given simultaneously with MCV4 (specially Menectra®) and CDC recommends at least one month interval between these two vaccines, with PCV13 given first.

10. **Whether any pre-exposure prophylaxis is needed for laboratory or health workers, routinely exposed to meningococcal infections?**

These cases may be given single dose of MCV4, followed by booster every 5 years, if exposure continues.

Key points

- **Vaccine:** Polysaccharide (MPSV) and Conjugate (MCV) vaccines

- **Dose:** 0.5 ml/dose over thigh/deltoid, SC (MPSV) or IM (MCV)

- **Schedule:** Not for Routine immunization, Only to High-risk cases –

  - *MPSV:* Single dose after 2 years of age, repeat once after 3-5 years

  - *MCV:* Single dose after 2 years of age,
        Booster after 5 year, if required (after 3 years till 7 years of age)
        (Two doses at 0, 3 mo in children aged 9-23 mo during outbreak/contact)

- **Efficacy** >85% (MPSV), 96-100% (MCV4)

- **Safety:** Side-effects rare except local reaction or transient mild fever, and

  - MPSV: Gastrointestinal upset, Myalgia, Regional lymphadenopathy

  - MCV4: Guillaine Barre syndrome (GBS)

- **Contraindications:** Past history of GBS (for MCV vaccine only)

References

1. World Health Organization. Meningococcal A conjugate vaccines: Position paper update: Weekly Epid Record 2015;90: 57-68.
2. Pemde HK. Meningococcal vaccines. *In:* IAP Guidebook on Immunization 2018-19 - Advisory Committee on Vaccines and Immunization Practices, Indian Academy of Pediatrics, 3rd Edition, New Delhi, Jaypee Brothers 2020; pp 352-366.
3. Mehta P. Meningococcal vaccines In: Vashishtha V et al. FAQs on Vaccines and immunization practices. 2nd Edition. .New Delhi, Jaypee Brothers 2015; pp 313-316.

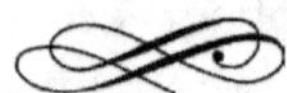

Cholera Vaccines

Cholera has caused many long pandemics in different parts of the world with very high mortality. Latest seventh pandemic, started in 1964, is still active. In India, disease is endemic throughout the country, with intermittent localized outbreaks.

Epidemiology: Cholera is caused by different strains of *vibrio cholerae 01*, a gram-negative motile bacteria with two major biotypes—*classical and eltor*, and many serotypes *(serovars)* according to somatic (O) antigens - mainly the *ogawa, inaba* and *hikojima* strains. Current infections in India are mainly caused by *eltor* biotype and *ogawa* serotypes. Last decade has seen emergence of a new virulent strain, i.e. *V. cholerae 0139* from Chennai.

The source of infection is either an asymptomatic carrier or a case, and infection is transmitted feco-oral route after ingestion of contaminated water or food. Children have the highest attack rate and more severe disease than in adults. Outbreaks usually begin in summer or rainy season or after large congregations of the people e.g. Kumbh mela.

After an incubation period of 12 hours to 5 days, ingested organisms colonize the epithelium and release a toxin, responsible for massive loss of intravascular and extracellular fluids and electrolytes.

Vaccines: Two whole-cell killed oral cholera vaccines are available in the world – a monovalent (Dukoral®) vaccine, containing *V cholera O1* with recombinant β subunit of cholera toxoid; and a bivalent vaccine containing *V. cholerae*

O1 (classic and El Tor) and *V. cholerae* O139, serotypes. Only bivalent vaccine (Shancol®) is licensed in India and discussed here. Phenol-inactivated whole cell vaccine, used earlier, has been discontinued due to higher side-effects and poor efficacy.

Contents & storage: Shancol® is available as single-dose ready-to use liquid formulation containing 600 Elisa units each of *O1 Inaba E1 Tor strain Phil 6973* and *O139 strain 4260B* and 300 Elisa units each of *O1 Ogawa classical strain Cairo 50*, O1 *Ogawa classical strain Cairo 50* and O1 *Inaba classical strain Cairo 48*, suspended in buffer solution. Vaccine contains Thiomersal and has a shelf life of 2 years at 2–8°C.

Dosage & administration: Shanchol® is given as 1.5 ml/dose orally.

Immunization Schedule: Cholera vaccine is not in NIS though its inclusion in highly endemic region, specially Bengal and Orissa, is under consideration. IAP recommends its use only in individuals residing in or travelling to highly endemic area or in high-risk circumstances for an outbreak e.g. Kumbh fair. WHO recommends that cholera vaccines should be used pre-emptively in endemic areas and in crises situations and not as outbreak control measure.

Shancol® is a two-dose vaccine, given at 2 weeks interval after one year of age, Booster dose is recommended after 2 years in cases with continued exposure.

Efficacy: Shancol® acts locally to induce an IgA antibody response, which prevents attachment of organisms to the gut receptors. Seroconversion rate, defined as four-fold rise in serum vibriocidal antibodies, is reported to be higher in children than in adults (80% vs 53%) and higher for Ogawa and Inaba serotypes (~70%) than for O139 strain (~20-60%).

Protection begins ~2 week after the second dose, with protective efficacy of ~65% for upto 3 years. Immunity wanes gradually and a booster dose is recommended after 2 years, if required.

Shancol® as a programmatic vaccine to control stable endemic cholera disease has shown an efficacy of 69% and 53% in Bangladesh.

Safety: Adverse events are rare except mild gastrointestinal upset e.g. Diarrhea, Vomiting or Abdominal pain. Fever, itching and dryness of mouth have been reported.

Contraindications include hypersensitivity to any vaccine component or after previous dose. Vaccination may be delayed during acute gastrointestinal or febrile illness, but not for minor illnesses. Vaccine may not be taken up appropriately in Immunocompromised persons, and if possible, vaccination must be postponed till completion of immunosuppressive treatment.

Frequently Asked Questions (FAQs)

1. **Who should receive the Cholera vaccine?**

   IAP recommends it only to individuals residing in or travelling to highly endemic area or in high-risk circumstances for an outbreak e.g. Kumbh fair. WHO recommends its use pre-emptively in endemic areas and cholera vaccine is under consideration for inclusion in national program for High endemic regions e.g. Bengal and Orissa.

2. **Whether Cholera vaccine can be used to control outbreaks?**

   It should not be used as an outbreak control measure as it is a two-dose vaccine and protection begins only after about 2 weeks of the second dose.

3. Whether this vaccine prevents other types of diarrhea?

No. however, another cholera vaccine Dukoral®, which is not marketed in India, offers some cross-protection against Enterotoxigenic *E. coli* infections.

4. Whether Booster dose is required?

Protective immunity wanes gradually and a booster dose is recommended after 2 years only in individuals who continue to reside in the highly endemic area.

Key points

- **Vaccine:** Whole cell Killed, bivalent, single-dose Liquid formulation.

- **Dose:** PO 1.5 ml/ dose

- **Schedule:** Indicated only for high-risk population or before Expected outbreak-conditions e.g. large fairs.

  Two doses at 2-week interval after infancy, Booster after 2 years if required.

- **Efficacy:** ~65% for 3 years, relatively less for O139 strain and in adults.

- **Safety:** Side-effects rare, except mild gastrointestinal upset.

- **Contraindications:** None, defer during diarrhea, febrile illness and immunosuppressive therapy.

References

1. World Health Organization. Cholera vaccines: Position paper: Weekly Epid Record 2017;92:477-500.
2. Guduru VK. Cholera vaccines: *In*: IAP Guidebook on Immunization 2018-19 - Advisory Committee on Vaccines and Immunization Practices, Indian Academy of Pediatrics, 3rd Edition, New Delhi, Jaypee Brothers 2020; pp 382-386.
3. Gangulu N. Cholera Vaccines. *In:* Vashishtha V et al. FAQs on Vaccines and immunization practices. 2nd Edition. New Delhi, Jaypee Brothers 2015; pp 317-322.
4. Clemens JD et al. Cholera vaccines. *In:* Plotkin S et al. (Eds). Plotkin's Vaccines, 7th ed. New York: Elsevier; 2017; pp. 185-6.

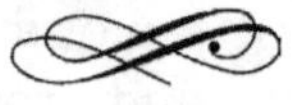

Rabies Vaccines

Rabies is a preventable but nearly always fatal CNS infection with India accounting for over half of the total world cases. Recent years have seen a spurt in dog population, dog bites and rabies deaths in many states. WHO has endorsed a target of *Zero Human Rabies Deaths* from dog-transmitted rabies by 2030.

Epidemiology: Rabies is a zoonosis caused by a neurotropic RNA virus *Lyssavirus seortype 1* present in saliva of infected animal e.g. dogs, cats and wild canines; and transmitted via bites, scratches, and licks on the mucous membrane or non-intact skin. Dog bites account for >96% cases of human rabies in India, followed by cats (2%). Human-to-human transmission is extremely rare, reported only via organ transplants.

After inoculation with contaminated saliva, virus replicates in local soft tissue and unless neutralized immunologically, irreversibly gets attached to the peripheral nerves. At this stage, disease becomes inevitable as virus spreads within neuronal sheaths towards brain to cause encephalitis with nearly universal fatality. Incubation period usually averages 4–6 weeks, but may range from 5 days to 6 years.

Maximum cases of dog bites occur in school-children, specially boys, due to their outdoor life style. Limited Indian data suggests that most rabies deaths also occur in children <15 years (50%), males (62%), and rural areas (91%). In India, *union territories of Lakshadweep and Andaman/Nicobar islands* are free from this disease.

Vaccines: Currently, two types of anti-rabies vaccines (ARVs) are available in India—

a) Cell-culture vaccines, e.g. Purified chick-embryo vaccine (PCEV), Human diploid-cell vaccine (HDCV), Purified Vero-cell vaccines (PVRV).

b) Embryonated egg-based vaccines e.g. Purified duck-embryo vaccine (PDEV).

Contents & storage: All ARVs contain minimum 2.5 IU antigen/dose as per WHO recommendation, though they differ with each other on the basis of viral strains and methodology to grow and inactivate virus. PCEV uses *Flury LEP-25* strain grown on chick fibroblasts(Rabipur®, Vaxirab-N®), HDCV uses *Pitman-Moore L503* or *Flury* strain grown on MRC-5 human diploid cells (Imovax-Rabies®), PVRV uses *Wistar* strain grown on Vero cells cultures (Abhayrab®, Verorab®, Rabivax-S®, Indirab®) and PDEV uses *Pittman Moore strain* grown on duck embryo cells (Vaxirab®).

All ARVs are supplied in lyophilized form with sterile water as diluents. These vaccines need to be stored at 2-8°C. Reconstituted vaccines should be used within 8 hours, if being used intradermally in more than one patient.

Dosage & administration: ARVs can be given intramuscularly or intradermally (except HDCV).

Generally, all ARVs are to be given after reconstitution as 1 ml/dose (except PVRV as 0.5 ml/dose) intramuscularly over upper arm or anterolateral thigh (children <2 years). *Rabies vaccines should never be injected in the gluteal region.*

PVRV/PCEV vaccines (not HDCV) can also be given intradermally as 0.1 ml/dose, irrespective of the reconstituted volume (differs for PVRV as 0.5 ml and PCEV as 1ml) at same sites, using disposable 1 ml syringe, preferably with fixed 28 G needle. Syringes with detachable needles are not preferred due to wastage of vaccine.

Immunization schedule varies with the purpose of vaccination (Post-exposure or Pre-exposure prophylaxis) and the route of immunization (Intramuscular or intradermal), as follows –

Intramuscular Post-exposure prophylaxis (IM-PEP): WHO (2018) recommends following options for IM-PEP using total four IM doses of any ARV vaccine, with day '0' being the day of commencement of vaccination, as soon as possible after exposure.

a) *Standard regimen* of total four doses of IM-ARV on days 0,3,7 and between day 14-28, also recommended by IAP and Government of India.

b) *Zagreb schedule,* with two dose of IM-ARV on day 0 (both deltoids) and one dose IM-ARV on days 7 and 21, needs one less visit, but not licensed in India.

Conventional Five-dose *Essen protocol* (IM D 0,3,7,14,28) is no longer considered necessary.

An additional dose on day 90 is optional and may be offered to those with immunocompromized state or severe disability (IAP).

Intradermal Post-exposure prophylaxis (ID-PEP) is cost-effective alternative to intramuscular vaccination due to lesser dose (0.1 ml) requirement, when large numbers of vaccinees are available simultaneously e.g. in major public health centers. ID vaccination is not recommended for individual practice, in immunocompromised cases or in those on chloroquine therapy. Only PVRV or PCEV vaccines (Not HDCV) can be used ID, given as 0.1 ml/dose. Drug Controller General of India has approved ID-PEP in large government anti-rabies centers with minimum 50 patients per day, using PVRV.

For ID-PEP, recommended regimens are –

a) Regimen used in National Rabies prophylaxis program, with two ID doses at different sites on day 0, 3, 7 and 28 (similar to updated Thai Red-cross regimen)

b) Shorter One week Two-site ID regimen, given on days 0, 3 and 7, also recommended by the WHO (2018) and IAP.

Thai Red-Cross Regimen (2-2-2-0-1-1) with two-site ID doses on days 0, 3, 7 and single dose on day 30 and 90 continues to be used in some countries.

Re-exposure prophylaxis: Immunological memory after PEP last for 5-21 years and previously vaccinated cases show good anamnestic responses on re-exposure even when antibodies are no longer detectable. Recommended PEP on re-exposure is as follows –

- No PEP is recommended in cases with re-exposure within 3 months of completion of previous PEP, except local wound care;

- For re-exposure after >3 months of full PEP/PrEP, only two booster doses are recommended on day 0 and 3, given intramuscularly or intradermally. Some workers advise additional dose on Day 7, if >10 years have lapsed.

- If second visit is not possible, as in case of travelers, a single-visit 4-site ID booster injections (two deltoids and two suprascapular region) may be given as per WHO recommendation.

- Rabies immunoglobulin is not advised on re-exposure as it may inhibit the anamnestic response.

- In cases with incomplete or undocumented PEP during previous exposure, complete PEP, discussed earlier, is recommended

Pre-exposure prophylaxis (PrEP) is recommended for occupationally high-risk population frequently exposed to animals e.g. Veterinarians, Laboratory-workers dealing with virus research or vaccine manufacture, Zoo/Forest-workers, Dog-catchers, Postmen, courier boys etc. It may also be considered to travelers to endemic regions with extensive outdoor activities. PrEP is generally not needed in children, though IAP recommends it after discussion with parents, specially in those who are exposed to pets at home or at higher risk of dog bites. WHO recommends PrEP in rabies endemic areas with dog-bite incidence of > 5% per year.

PrEP regimen include two doses of any vaccine - either single-site IM or Two-site ID on day 0 and 7, recommended by WHO and IAP. In National rabies prophylaxis program, total three doses of IM/ID vaccine are used for PrEP, on day 0, 7 and 21/28.

Routine assessment of antibody titers after vaccination is not recommended except in immunocompromised cases, though it is advisable to monitor antibody titers every 6-12 months in those with frequent exposure and give a booster dose, if titers fall <0.5 IU/ml. If serologic testing is not available, booster vaccination every 5 years is advised.

Efficacy: ARVs largely protect through T-cell dependent Neutralizing antibodies against G-proteins, though cell-mediated immunity also plays some role. Post-vaccination, serum vaccine-induced neutralizing antibody (VNA) titers above 0.5 IU/mL are considered as protective.

All ARVs are equally immunogenic, achieving protective serological titers in > 99% vaccinees following PEP/PrEP. Appropriate PEP along with proper wound management and simultaneous administration of RIG is almost invariably effective in preventing rabies. Immunological memory last for 5-21 years after primary series and previously vaccinated cases show good anamnestic responses after booster doses even when antibodies are no longer detectable.

Safety: Side-effects are uncommon except transient local reactions e.g. pain, swelling and pruritus and mild systemic reactions e.g. fever, headache, dizziness and gastrointestinal upset. Local reactions are more common with Intradermal vaccination versus intramuscular route.

Side effects are more common with HDCV (20-70%) than other CCV vaccines (2-7%). Transient immune complex-like reactions presenting with urticaria, arthralgia, angioedema etc. have been reported with HDCV, specially after booster doses, generally attributed to the stabilizer used in the vaccine - Human albumin. Few cases resembling transient Guillain-Barre syndrome have been also reported with HDCV, though cause-effect relationship is uncertain.

Contraindications: Considering the near fatality of rabies disease, there is no contraindication for ARVs including infancy, pregnancy, lactation or concurrent illnesses. PCEV should be avoided in children with history of egg-allergy.

Frequently Asked Questions (FAQs)

1. **Which vaccine is preferable for ARV vaccinations?**

   All available ARV vaccines have standard antigenic content (2.5 IU/dose) and are equally immunogenic and protective. However, HDCV is not approved for ID-PEP and has higher incidence of local and systemic side effects.

2. **Whether IM route is preferable over ID route for PEP?**

   ID-PEP is the cost-effective alternative to intramuscular vaccination due to lesser dose (0.1 ml) requirement, with comparable protective efficacy. However, it is worthwhile only if large number of vaccinees are available simultaneously, as in major public health centers. ID vaccination is not recommended for individual practice, in immunocompromised cases or in those on chloroquine therapy.

3. **Whether switch-over from ID to IM route or vice versa is permitted?**

   Switch over from IM to ID or ID to IM route of admin-istration during PEP is not recommended due to lack of sufficient immunogenicity data following such change.

However, if unavoidable, there is no need to re-start the schedule and doses taken by the earlier route must be considered as valid.

4. **Whether ARV vaccine brands can be changed for subsequent doses, if the brand used in previous dose/s is not available?**

Interchange of vaccine is not advisable, permitted only if unavoidable.

5. **What should be done if a PEP dose was missed or delayed after initiation?**

In cases of any missed/delayed dose, re-initiation is not required and vaccination can be resumed as though the patient was on schedule, maintaining the same interval between doses. For example, if dose 3 was given on D10 (rather than D7), dose 4 must be given on D17-31 instead of D14-28.

6. **Is it mandatory to continue PEP if the animal is alive and well after 10 days?**

In case of IM-PEP, further doses may be skipped if the animal remains healthy till 10 days after bite, though, course should be completed in case of ID-PEP, irrespective of status of animal.

Moreover, observation period of 10 days is valid for dogs and cats only. Natural history of rabies in other mammals is not fully understood and such animal bites should receive full PEP.

7. **Whether PEP is needed after bite by a pet dog?**

In case of bites by pet animals, PEP must be started immediately, irrespective of the prior vaccination status of the animal since animal vaccine failures are known due to improper administration, poor quality of vaccine and poor health status of animal. Further, the vaccine induced protection to animal may not always be long-lasting.

8. **Whether a person needs PEP if presents after 3 months of dog bite?**

   All persons presenting several days/ months/ years after the bite should be managed as the person who was bitten recently as rabies has a long incubation period.

   However, likelihood of developing rabies declines progressively, with risk being negligible after 12 months. If vaccine supply is limited, vaccine can therefore be reserved for suspect and probable rabies exposures that occurred recently or within 12 months.

9. **Whether PEP needs to be repeated on re-exposure?**

   Re-exposure prophylaxis is recommended if more than 3 months have lapsed since last PEP/PrEP dose taken previously as follows –

   a) In fully pre-vaccinated cases (PrEP/PEP), only two doses are recommended on day 0 and 3 of exposure given intramuscularly or intradermally (Two-site on each day). If second visit is not possible e.g. in travelers, single-visit 4-site ID booster injections (two deltoids and two suprascapular region) may be given as per WHO recommendation. Some workers advise additional dose on Day 7, if >10 years have lapsed.

   b) Complete 4-dose IM/ID PEP is recommended in cases with incomplete or undocumented PEP following previous exposure.

      Rabies immunoglobulin is not advised on re-exposure as it may inhibit the anamnestic response.

9. **What should be the PEP after a dog bite in HIV infected person?**

   Patients with HIV/AIDS and low CD4 counts (< 200 cells/ mm^3 or < 25% in children < 5 years) may not develop sufficient antibody response after ARV. In them, as well as in others with significant immunosuppression including chemotherapy or prolonged steroid therapy, thorough wound management along with RIG is essential even for category II bites, apart from PEP via intramuscular route only. It is preferable to assess serum VNA titers after 10 days of the last ARV dose, to ensure appropriate protection.

10. Which animal bites are considered potentially risky for Rabies?

Bites by any warm-blooded animal, including dogs, cats, cattle, pigs, donkeys, horses and wild animals are potentially risky. In India, 97% rabies cases are due to dog bites followed by cats (2%), jackals, mongoose and others (1%). All bites by all wild animals or animals in the forest should be treated as category III exposure. Bat rabies is unknown in India and at present, exposure to bats here does not warrant PEP.

All dog bites are considered as potential risk for rabies even if it was unprovoked or the dog is domestic and vaccinated.

11. Whether PEP is required after Rodent bite?

Rabies due to domestic rodent bites, squirrel etc has not been reported in India and PEP is not normally recommended for these bites. However, PEP is advisable following bite by wild rodents.

12. Whether PEP is required in close contacts or health workers after exposure to a human rabies case?

Human-to-human transmission is almost unknown except few cases due to infected corneal transplant. However, people who have been exposed closely to the secretions of a patient with rabies may be offered PEP as a precautionary measure. (National guidelines, 2019)

13. What are the current guidelines for management of a dog-bite?

A classification system, depending on the severity of exposure and risk of disease is frequently used to

Category	Exposure	Local wound care	RIG/ RMA	ARV
I	• Licks on unbroken skin • Touching/feeding of animals	Yes	No	No
II	• Nibbling of uncovered skin • Minor scratches, no bleeding • Licks on broken skin	Yes	No	Yes
III	• Single/multiple transdermal bites Licks over broken skin or mucous membranes	Yes	Yes	Yes

Table 23.1: WHO Categories for exposure risk and PEP after Dog bite

RIG: Rabies Immunoglobulin or Monoclonal Antibody),
ARV: Anti rabies vaccine

decide needs for post-exposure prophylaxis (**Table 23.1**). Important steps in the management of a dog-bite include -(a) Local wound care, (b) passive immunization (d) active immunization.

14. What is the role of local wound care in PEP?

Local wound care is essential in all cases presenting soon after bite, including category I bites, to kill the virus by mechanical and virucidal action. Proper wound care reduces risk of rabies by 80% and involves immediate washing of wounds, even licks, and adjoining area with soap and running water for 15 minutes. Deep wounds need to be irrigated with virucidal agents, e.g. povidone iodine or 70% alcohol. Antimicrobials and Tetanus toxoid should be given, if indicated.

Suturing of the wounds must be avoided as further trauma increases local vascularity and facilitates spread of virus in deep tissues. If essential, temporary stay sutures may be applied after local infiltration of RIG, followed by regular suturing after 48 hours.

15. Which cases of animal bite need passive immunization?

Passive immunization aims to prevent immediate attachment of virus to the nerve endings till vaccine-induced immunity develops. It is recommended for - *a) All category III bites, b) Category II and III bites in immunocompromized persons, or c) All bites by wild animals.* It is most effective when given immediately after exposure, but may be given till 7th day of first vaccine dose, by which the active immune response to vaccine is expected to develop. Passive immunization is not advised on re-exposure in previously vaccinated cases, as it may inhibit the anamnestic response.

16. What are different options for passive immunization and which one is preferable?

Presently, there are three options for Passive immunization - Human rabies immunoglobulin (HRIG), Equine rabies immunoglobulin (ERIG) and Monoclonal Antibodies (MAb)). WHO as well as IAP encourages use of monoclonal antibodies instead of RIG due to easier availability, lower cost, lesser side effects, and possibly greater effectiveness.

17. *Which monoclonal antibody products are available in India and how should they be given?*

Monoclonal antibodies bind ectodomain of G glycoprotein of the virus to block its entry into neighboring cells, currently available as two products - *Rabishield®* containing Recombinant human monoclonal bodies and Twinrab®, a cocktail of two *murine* monoclonal antibodies - Docaravimab and Miromavimab. Both products are nearly comparable in efficacy and cost, though former is more economical. These antibodies must be infiltrated locally at the time of the first vaccine dose or upto 7th day of first dose. If the calculated dose is insufficient to infiltrate all the wounds, it may be diluted in sterile normal saline to get a volume enough to be infiltrated around all the wounds.

Rabishield® is available 40 IU/ml, with recommended dose of 3.3 IU/kg, Twinrab® is available as 300 or 600 IU/ml with recommended dose of 40 IU/Kg.

18. How should the Rabies immunoglobulins (RIG) be given in category III bites?

Two types of Rabies immunoglobulins are available – a) Human rabies immunoglobulin (150 IU/ml) which is preferable and safer but costly, and b) Equine anti-rabies serum (300 IU/ml), which is relatively cheap but carries a small risk of anaphylaxis (1/1,50,000) or serum sickness. Recommended dose for HRIG is 20 IU/kg (max1500 IU), while ERIG doses are double of that i.e. 40 IU/kg (max 3000 IU).

RIG must be infiltrated into and around the wound with maximum quantity that is anatomically feasible, even if the wound is infected. For large and multiple wounds, it can be diluted with physiological buffer saline to ensure the infiltration of all wounds. However, total dose of RIG must not exceed the recommended one, as it may suppress the antibody production following ARV. *WHO no longer recommends injecting remainder of the calculated RIG dose intramuscularly away from the wound.*

RIG is safe except local tenderness and mild fever. It is important to avoid and recognize the *compartment syndrome* which occurs if large volumes of RIG are injected into a small body area with limited tissue.

19. Whether Skin testing is required before ERIG due to potential risk of anaphylaxis?

WHO does not recommend skin testing prior to ERIG administration as skin tests do not accurately predict anaphylaxis risk and ERIG should be given irrespective of the result due to urgency of passive immunization, if alternative is not available. Most of the new ERIG preparations are potent, safe, highly purified and carry a small risk of anaphylaxis.

20. Can same RIG vial be used in multiple patients, considering the cost?

Calculated RIG dose can be fractionated in smaller, individual syringes to be used for several patients. However, it requires handling and storage in aseptic conditions. Unused fractionated doses and open vials of RIG should be discarded by the end of the day.

20. What are the advantages of pre-exposure prophylaxis?

Pre-exposure prophylaxis (PrEP) is important in persons with high risk of exposure risk, which is often unrecognized (health/laboratory workers) or unreported (children). PrEP eliminates the need for costly passive immunization and reduces PEP to two doses only.

21. Is there any alternative of passive immunization, if not available?

If RIG is not available, then two doses of the vaccine may be given on day 0. However, it is not a substitute for RIG Intradermal vaccination.

22. A person has received only single dose for PrEP. Is it protective?

While one dose of PrEP may confer some protection, it may not be enough. Such cases should receive the second dose as soon as possible and within 1 year. They need full PEP, if exposed prior to the second dose, including RIG.

23. Whether PrEP boosters are needed in persons with continuous occupational exposure or living in high-risk area?

PrEP booster/s following a primary series of PrEP or PEP are not required for individuals with continuous exposure risk, unless immunocompromized, who need to monitor antibody titers every 6-12 months and receive a booster dose, if titers fall <0.5 IU/ml. In case the serologic testing is not available, booster vaccination every 5 years is advised in these cases.

> **Key points**
>
> - **Vaccine:** Cell-culture vaccines (PCEV, HDCV, PVRV) or Embryonated egg-based vaccines (PDEV).
> - **Dose:** IM 1.0 ml (0.5 ml for PVRV) *or* ID 0.1 ml (HDCV not used ID)
> - **Immunization Schedules:**
>   *Post-exposure:* Total four IM doses on D 0,3,7 & 14-21, or
>   Total six ID doses, Two per visit on different sites on D 0,3 & 7.
>   *Re-exposure:* Total two IM or ID doses on day 0 & 7, if >3 mo have lapsed
>   *Pre-exposure:* Total two doses of 1-site IM or 2-site ID on day 0 & 7.
> - **Efficacy:** All vaccines are equally immunogenic (> 99%)
> - **Safety:** Local reactions more common with ID injections, Transient Fever/Headache (More common with HDCV), sp Allergy and GBS?
> - **Contraindications**: None, PCEV may be avoided in H/O severe egg allergy
>
> **Note**: Passive immunization, preferably with monoclonal antibodies is recommended, in all class III bites, Class III & II bites in immunocompromised persons and all bites by wild animals, but not on re-exposure among previously vaccinated cases.

References

1. World Health Organization. Rabies vaccines: Position paper: Weekly Epid. Record 2018;93:201-220.
2. National centre for disease control. National Guidelines on Rabies Prophylaxis. Available at *https://ncdc.gov.in/WriteReadData/linkimages/NationalGuidelinesforRabiesprophylaxis2019.pdf2015.* (accessed on 21st July 2021).
3. Guduru VK. Rabies Vaccines: *In*: IAP Guidebook on Immunization 2018-19 - Advisory Committee on Vaccines and Immunization Practices, Indian Academy of Pediatrics, 3rd Edition, New Delhi, Jaypee Brothers 2020; pp 367-381.
4. Choudhury J. Rabies *In:* Vashishtha V et al. FAQs on Vaccines and immunization practices. 2nd Edition. New Delhi, Jaypee Brothers 2015; pp 239-253.

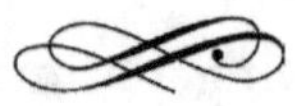

Yellow Fever Vaccine

Yellow fever, though confined only to some countries in sub-Saharan Africa and Central/South America, is a serious vector-borne illness with clinical spectrum spanning from mild influenza-like illness to severe hepatitis and hemorrhagic fever.

Epidemiology: Yellow fever virus is RNA virus, present in the infected humans from just before the onset of fever to first 3–5 days of illness, and transmitted via the bite of infected mosquito, primarily *Aedes aegypti.* Disease does not exist in India, though conditions here are conducive for its spread due to the presence of the vector *Aedes aegypti* and favorable environment. Risk for a traveller to the endemic area is estimated to be ~25-350/100,000/week. Government of India has strict regulations in place to restrict the entry of susceptible and unvaccinated individuals from endemic countries.

Vaccine: Yellow fever vaccine (YFV) is a live attenuated vaccine derived from 17D strain of the virus grown on chick140 embryo cells. It is the only commercially available vaccine against yellow fever.

Contents & Storage: YFV is available as a freeze-dried preparation in single/multi-dose vials along with sterile saline as diluent. Vaccine must be stored at 2-8°C. Reconstituted vaccine is heat labile and must be used within one hour.

Dose & administration: YFV is given as 0.5 ml/dose of reconstituted vaccine subcutaneously or intramuscularly.
Immunization Schedule: In India, YFV is recommended

only to the travelers going to notified endemic countries (FAQ1), as single dose, preferably at least 10 days before the travel.

In endemic countries, it is recommended as routine immunization at 9-12 months of age. Vaccine is not recommended below 9 months except during epidemics and it is contraindicated below six months of age.

Efficacy: Immunogenicity and efficacy of YFV is above 90%, relatively less in pregnancy and immunocompromized states. Protection begins after 10th day of vaccination and lasts life-long.

Safety: Vaccine is very safe though 10–30% recipients report systemic side effects e.g. mild fever, headache, and myalgia for 5-10 days. Severe adverse reactions are rare and include allergic reactions e.g. urticaria, bronchospasm or very rarely anaphylaxis (1.8/ lac doses), specially in persons with egg allergy.

Other rare (<1/lac doses) but important adverse events include –

a) *Yellow fever vaccine-associated neurologic disease (YELAND),* presenting as meningoencephalitis, Guillain-Barré syndrome, acute disseminated encephalomyelitis or bulbar/facial palsy, after 3-28 days of vaccination, more common in elderly people; and

b) *Yellow fever vaccine-associated viscerotropic disease (YELAVD), a severe* illness mimicking wild disease after 1-8 days of vaccination with multisystem organ failure and death.

While YELAND is rarely fatal, case fatality rate of YELAVD is ~65%. Both complications are more common in first time vaccinees and in persons > 60 years.

Contraindications: YF vaccine is contraindicated in infants

<6 months, or those with history of thymus disease, severely immunocompromised state including HIV with CD4 count < 15% and history of serious egg allergy. Vaccine must be avoided in infants aged 6–9 months, individuals > 65 years and pregnant or lactating women.

Frequently Asked Questions (FAQs)

1. **Who should receive Yellow fever vaccine in India?**

   In India, Yellow fever vaccination is recommended only for travel to endemic and transitional areas as per International Health Regulations. Following countries are regarded as endemic, for which vaccination is required -

   Africa: Angola, Bénin, Burkina Faso, Burundi, Cameroon, Central African Republic, Chad, Congo, Côte d'Ivoire, Democratic Republic of the Congo, Equatorial Guinea, Ethiopia, Gabon, The Gambia, Ghana, Guinea, Guinea-Bissau, Kenya, Liberia, Mali, Niger, Nigeria, Rwanda, Senegal, Sierra Leone, Sudan, Togo, and Uganda.

   America: Bolivia, Brazil, Colombia, Ecuador, French Guiana, Guyana, Panama, Peru, Suriname, Trinidad and Tobago, and Venezuela.

2. **Where is the Yellow fever vaccine available for Travellers?**

   Yellow fever is generally available at health centers on international exit points like airports and ports. Nowadays, it can also be taken at select government designated centers in large cities.

3. **What is International certificate of vaccination or prophylaxis (ICVP)?**

   All Yellow fever vaccinees receive an *international certificate of vaccination or prophylaxis* (ICVP), duly dated, stamped and signed by the center administering the vaccine, valid after 10ᵗʰ day of vaccination.

4. **A person, who received YFV 15 years back will be travelling again to an endemic country. Whether he needs re-vaccination?**

    ICVP validity has been extended life-long w.e.f. 11ᵗʰ july 2016 and no revaccination is required regardless of the date of vaccination.

5. **What will happen if a person travels without ICVP?**

    In absence of ICVP, the traveller may be quarantined, denied entry or revaccinated at the point of entry to a country, though last one is not a recommended option.

    In India, any traveller > 9 months of age, arriving by air or sea from notified high-risk countries without ICVP is detained in isolation for up to 6 days if s/he -

    - arrives within 6 days of departure from an high-risk area,

    - has been in such an area in transit (except if remained in the airport during entire stay and the health officer agrees to such an exemption),

    - arrives on a ship that started/ touched a high-risk area up to 30 days before its arrival in India, unless it has been disinfected with WHO-recommended procedures.

    - arrives on an aircraft, which has been in a high-risk area, unless it has been disinfected with WHO-recommended procedures.

6. **What should the travelers with a contraindication for yellow fever vaccinations do?**

    In case of medical contraindications mentioned earlier (infants <6 months, Thymic disease, severe immunodeficiency, serious egg allergy) physician must issue a signed waiver in ICVP, though such waiver does not guarantee its acceptance by the destination country.

> **Key points**
>
> - **Vaccine:** Live attenuated, Lyophilized vaccine
>
> - **Dose:** 0.5 ml / dose given SC/IM after reconstitution with diluent
>
> - **Schedule:** Single dose, only to travelers to endemic country, at least 10 days before travel.
>
> - **Protective Efficacy** *:* > 90%, Life-long.
>
> - **Side effects:** *Common:* Mild fever, headache, myalgia for 5-10 days
>
>   *Rare:* Allergic reactions, YELAND, YELAVD (see text)
>
> - **Contraindications:** Age <6 mo or >65 years, Pregnancy or lactation Thymus disease, Egg allergy, Immunodeficiency states.

References

1. Guduru VK. Yellow Fever vaccine.: *In:* IAP Guidebook on Immunization 2018-19 - Advisory Committee on Vaccines and Immunization Practices, Indian Academy of Pediatrics, 3rd Edition, New Delhi, Jaypee Brothers 2020; pp 387-395.
2. World Health Organization. New yellow fever vaccination requirements for travelers. Available from *https://www.who.int/ith/updates/20160727/en/* [accessed 16th May 2021].

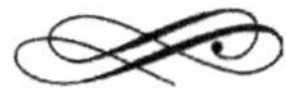

Section

V

Vaccines Under Development

Newer (Pipeline) Vaccines

As of today, vaccines against 26 diseases are available for clinical use globally and recommended by the WHO in all or selected populations, latest being Covid-19 vaccines. Another over 500 vaccines against many more diseases are in different stages of development or trial phase, often referred as *Pipeline vaccines*.

The term Newer vaccines is not well defined though may be interpreted as the vaccines which are still in trial phase and not available for regular use. These include either alternatives to the existing vaccines e.g. BCG, *or* the vaccines against the diseases for which no vaccine is available till date for clinical use.

Out of all the pipeline vaccines listed in **Table 25.1**, two products have been marketed commercially for limited use in some countries i.e. one for the Dengue fever and another for the malaria. One RSV vaccine candidate has reached the stage of phase III trial in pregnant women, aiming to transfer to the immunity to their offsprings for early protection. Another set of newer vaccines against Covid-19, discussed in Chapter 25, considering its relevance to present times.

Remaining newer vaccines, though offer exciting opportunities, are still in experimental phase or early trial stage and hence, not discussed in this practice-oriented book. Alternatives to existing vaccines, if available in other countries or in advanced stages of development, have been discussed in respective chapters.

Table 25.1: Currently Available and Pipeline (Newer) vaccines

Available vaccines	Pipeline vaccines
• Cholera	• Campylobacter jejuni
• COVID-19 (coronovairus)	• Chagas Disease
• Dengue	• Chikungunya
• Diphtheria	• Enterotoxigenic Escherichia coli
• Hepatitis A	• Enterovirus 71 (EV71)
• Hepatitis B	• Group B Streptococcus (GBS)
• *Haemophilus influenzae* type b (Hib)	• Herpes Simplex Virus
• Human papillomavirus (HPV)	• Hepatitis C
• Influenza	• Hepatitis E
• Japanese encephalitis	• HIV-1
• Malaria	• Human Hookworm Disease
• Measles	• Leishmaniasis Disease
• Meningococcal meningitis	• Malaria
• Mumps	• Neisseria gonorrhoeae
• Pertussis	• Nipah Virus
• Pneumococcal disease	• Nontyphoidal Salmonella Disease
• Poliomyelitis	• Norovirus
• Rabies	• Paratyphoid fever
• Rotavirus	• Respiratory Syncytial Virus (RSV)
• Rubella	• Schistosomiasis Disease
• Tetanus	• Shigella
• Tick-borne encephalitis	• Staphylococcus aureus
• Tuberculosis	• Streptococcus pneumoniae
• Typhoid	• Streptococcus pyogenes
• Varicella	• Tuberculosis
• Yellow Fever	• Universal Influenza vaccines

Source:
https://www.who.int/teams/immunization-vaccines-and-biologicals/diseases

25.1: DENGUE VACCINES

CYD-TDV (Denguvaxia®) is the first and only licensed vaccine against Dengue, being used in some endemic countries of Asia and Latin America. Several other candidates are under development including two more live attenuated (recombinant) tetravalent vaccines in Phase 3 trials. Following details pertain only to licensed CYD-TDV vaccine.

Contents & Storage: CYD-TDV is a live attenuated, recombinant tetravalent vaccine containing four recombinant dengue serotypes, each obtained separately by replacing the genes encoding the prM and E proteins of the attenuated YF 17D vaccine virus genome with the corresponding genes of the 4 wild dengue serotypes.

It is a freeze-dried single-dose or multi-dose formulation, to be reconstituted using 0.4% sodium chloride diluent (0.9% for multi-dose vials), before use. Lyophilized vaccine must be stored at 2-8°C and should be used within 6 hours of reconstitution, as it does not contain an preservative.

Immunization schedule includes total three doses of 0.5 ml subcutaneously, given at 6 months interval. While vaccine is licensed for use between 9-45 years of age, the optimal age of vaccination depends on local disease epidemiology (see WHO recommendations below).

Efficacy: Immunogenicity of the vaccine is higher in vaccinees who are seropositive to any serotype (i.e. had evidence of prior dengue infection) before vaccination than in baseline seronegative vaccinees.

Protective efficacy in trial participants aged 2-16 years was reported as 54.7% against serotype 1, 43.0% against serotype 2, 71.6% against serotype 3, and 76.9% against serotype 4. Efficacy against hospitalization due to dengue and severe dengue in the first 25 months was higher than efficacy in preventing symptomatic disease of any severity. Pooled vaccine efficacy against hospitalization and severe illness was 72.7% aand 79.1% respectively, being higher in older participants aged above 9 Years.

Safety: Side-effects include transient local reactions and minor systemic reactions e.g. Myalgia, Headache and malaise in about half of the cases.

However, it is very important to note that *outcome of CYD-TDV vaccination differs in seropositive and seronegative individuals at the time of vaccination. In seropositive individuals, the vaccine is efficacious and safe. In seronegative individuals, the vaccine confers a low level of protection during first 2 years but is later followed by an increased risk of hospitalized and severe dengue.*

In seronegative case, the vaccine acts as first infection, eliciting immune reponse. However, if the vaccinated case acquires a second infection by wild virus exposure, disease will be more severe and complicated with severe thrombocytopenia and plasma leakage, as in the case of second of two natural infections in unvaccinated individuals. WHO Global Advisory Committee on Vaccine Safety (GACVS) recommends that invidduaalss who have not been infected with wild dengue virus, i.e. who are seronegative, should not be vaccinated with CYD-TDV.

In a seropositive case, vaccine acts as second infection with a attenuated virus, thus offering the protection but without pathogenic complications.

Contraindications include - (1) individuals with a history of severe allergic reaction to any component of the dengue vaccine or after prior administration of the dengue vaccine or a vaccine containing the same components; (2) individuals with congenital or acquired immune deficiency involving cell-mediated immunity; (3) individuals with symptomatic HIV infection or with asymptomatic HIV infection with evidence of impaired immune function; (4) Pregnancy & Lactation.

WHO Recommendations: WHO suggests following issues to be considered while planning to include Dengue vaccine in immunization programs -

- CYD-TDV is an efficacious and safe vaccine in persons who had a dengue virus infection in the past (seropositive individuals), but carries an increased risk of severe dengue in those who experience their first natural dengue infection after vaccination (seronegative individuals).

- Countries should consider introduction of the dengue vaccine CYD-TDV *only* if the minimization of risk among seronegative individuals can be assured.

- For countries considering vaccination in dengue control program, *pre-vaccination screening* is the recommended strategy, followed by vaccination of *only* seropositive subjects.

- If pre-vaccination screening is not feasible, vaccination without individual screening could be considered in areas with seroprevalence rates of at least 80% by age 9 years.

- Vaccinees must be clearly communicated that - a) No pre-vaccine screening is fool proof and a false-seropositive person may get more serious disease after vaccination, if exposed again to a wild infection.

- Optimal Age of the vaccination must be decided according to local disease epidemiology, targeting the population at an age just before the highest risk of severe dengue disease. It is a trade-off between the population benefit conferred by vaccination and the enhanced risk experienced by a subset of seronegative vaccine recipients. Generally, Targeted age is usually lower in countries with high transmission and higher in countries with low transmission.

25.2: MALARIA VACCINE

More than thirty vaccines against falciparum malaria are at pre-clinical and clinical stages of evaluation, acting on different stages of the parasite - Pre-erythrocytic stage, Erythrocytic stage, and transmission-blocking (gametocyte) vaccines. No vaccine against P vivax has gone beyond the laboratory stage due to problems of *in vitro* parasite culture to identity synergistic antigens.

RTS,S (Mosquirix®) is the only vaccine against malaria licensed on pilot basis (2019) in three sub-Saharan African countries – Ghana, Kenya and Malawi, which has shown significant reduction in prevalence as well as severity of falciparum malaria. Following discussion pertains to RTS,S Vaccine only. As of now, this vaccine is available only in these three countries, on prescription. WHO has not yet recommended it for the large-scale use beyond the pilot program.

Contents & Storage: RTS,S is a pre-erythrocytic stage hybrid recombinant protein vaccine containing P. falciparum circumsporozoite protein fused with hepatitis B surface antigen This recombinant fusion protein (RTS) is expressed together with free hepatitis B surface antigen (S), to form RTS,S virus-like particles.

RTS,S is a freeze-dried powder, supplied with a diluent and needs to reconstituted just before the use. Vaccine must be stored at 2-8°C and should be used within 6 hours of reconstitution.

Immunization schedule: As of now, the vaccine has been used only in children aged 5–17 months, given as 0.5 ml IM with four dose schedule - three doses at one month interval, followed by a fourth dose after 18 months.

Efficacy: The vaccine induces Humoral as well as cellular response to prevent maturation and multiplication of sporozoites in liver. It has shown ~ 39% efficacy against the disease *per se* and 29% against the severe malaria on four years follow-up, along with significant reduction in hospitalizations and need for blood transfusions. Vaccine does not offer any protection against P vivax malaria.

Safety: Vaccine is well tolerated except local side effects and increased risk of febrile seizures within 7 days. Although there are some reports of meningitis and cerebral malaria, no causal link was established.

25.3: RESPIRATORY SYNCYTIAL VIRUS (RSV) VACCINE

RSV is one of the leading causes of viral respiratory infections in infants and toddlers as well as in elderly and immunocompromized persons. Vaccines against RSV primarily aim to prevent serious RSV-associated lower respiratory infections. No RSV vaccine is licensed at present, though many are in trial phase including particle-based vaccines, live attenuated vaccines, protein subunit vaccines or vector-based vaccines.

Major obstacles to develop a successful RSV vaccines include - a) the need to immunize at very early age (RSV disease is most common in young infants), when child may not be immunocompetent enough to respond well to vaccination, b) Existence of two antigenically distinct RSV groups - A and B; and c) Potential risk of disease enhancement, as was seen following administration of an early generation formalin-inactivated vaccine. Attempts to develop an RSV vaccine began in 1960s with an unsuccessful formalin-inactivated vaccine, which unfortunately lead to development of a vaccine associated enhanced respiratory disease with significant morbidity and mortality in trial subjects.

Presently, one vaccine candidate is in phase III trials in pregnant women, using a recombinant subunit pre-fusion

RSV antigen (RSVPreF3). Early phase data suggest rapid boosting of pre-existing immunity in pregnant women with about 14-fold rise in RSV-A and RSV-B neutralizing antibody titers after vaccination. Phase III study of this GSK3888550A vaccine has been started since November 2020 and aims to assess the effect of maternal immunization on mothers as well as on infants born to these vaccinated mothers, who may be protected during high-risk period of early infancy via transplacentally transferred antibodies. A similar study for direct vaccination of infants as well as high-risk elderly population, but with different vaccine candidates, is also expected to start soon.

In absence of an effective vaccine, a specific RSV-F protein inhibitor monoclonal antibody – Palivizumab (Synagis®) has been recommended to prevent serious RSV infections in high-risk children i.e. Preterm <35 weeks (up to 6 months of age), Bronchopulmonary dysplasia requiring medical treatment within previous 6 months (up to 24 months of age) and hemodynamically significant congenital heart disease (up to 24 months of age), given as monthly injections (50 mg/kg/dose IM)during the RSV season.

References

1. World Health Organization. Research and product development by disease. Available at *https://www.who.int/teams/immunization-vaccines-and-biologicals/diseases* (accessed on 16th July 2021).
2. World Health Organization. Dengue Vaccine: Position paper: Weekly Epid. Record 2018;93:457-476.
3. World Health Organization. The malaria vaccine implementation programme 2020. Available at *https://www.who.int/news-room/q-a-detail/malaria-vaccine-implementation-programme* (accessed on 20th June 2021).
4. Deshpande S. Future vaccines. *In:* IAP Guidebook on Immunization 2018-19 - Advisory Committee on Vaccines and Immunization Practices, Indian Academy of Pediatrics, 3rd Edition, New Delhi, Jaypee Brothers 2020; pp 444-464.

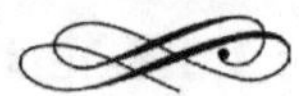

Corona virus disease 2019 (COVID-19) is a highly contagious disease caused by Severe acute respiratory syndrome coronavirus 2 (SARS-CoV-2), responsible for current global pandemic with over 217 million cases and 4.5 million death world-wide, including 32.8 million cases and 4.3 lac deaths in India (Till August 2021). First known case was identified in Wuhan, China in December 2019, while first Indian case was reported from Kerala on 27th January 2020.

Epidemiology: Corona virus is an enveloped positive-stranded RNA virus of same subgenus as the severe acute respiratory syndrome (SARS) virus and hence designated as (SARS-CoV-2. Transmitted largely person-to-person as a droplet infection, entered virus binds to the host receptor-Angiotensin converting enzyme-2 (ACE2) on the surface through receptor-binding domain of its spike protein to gain the entry and multiply intracellularly as well as infect other cells.

Like other viruses, SARS-CoV-2 too mutates frequently with no significant impact, though some variants have received widespread attention due to higher infectivity or morbidity, termed as *"variants of concern"*.

In India, SARS-CoV-2 Variant of B.1.617.2 lineage, commonly referred as Delta variant is major cause of concern due to higher infectivity and risk of hospitalization. Efficacy of available vaccines is another major concern in mutant viruses. However, recent studies suggest that though less effective, many of the presently used vaccines offer good protection against the Delta variant.

Immune responses following infection include both humoral SARS-CoV-2-specific antibodies as well as cell-mediated responses, which are protective though the duration of protection is unknown. Humoral response may be weak and short-lived after milder infections than after severe disease, though specific memory cells have been demonstrated in recovered patients suggestive of anamnestic response on re-infection.

Vaccine: Till August 2021, WHO has approved seven vaccines for global use (**Table 26.1**) of which only Pfizer-BioNTech's BNT162b2 vaccine has been granted full approval for persons above 16 years. Other vaccines have been approved under emergency use listing. AstraZeneca's AZD1222 is the highest distributed vaccine in the world, with 115 countries having recognized it.

Three of the WHO approved vaccines are not yet approved in India (Pfizer's, *BBIBP's & Sinovac's*). India has granted emergency use authorization to seven vaccines under till August 2021 (**Table 26.1**), some of whom are not yet approved by the WHO.

Table 26.1: WHO and India approved Covid-19 vaccines	
WHO Approved Covid Vaccines	**India Approved Covid vaccines**
• *Pfizer-BioNTech's* …. BNT162b2	• *Serum Institute of India's…* Covidshield®
• *Moderna's…..* mRNA1273	• *Bharat Biotech's….* Covaxin®
• *Johnson & Johnson's….* AD26.COV2.S	• *Gamaleya's….* SputunikV® (Dr Reddy's Lab)
• *Oxford-Astrazeneca's….* AZDI1222	• *Moderna's…* mRNA1273 (Cipla Lab),
• *Serum Institute of India's….* ChAdOx1	• *Johnson & Johnson's…* Janssen® (Biological E)
• *BBIP-Sinopharm's …..* BBIBP-CorV	• *Astrazeneca's….* AZDI1222
• *Sinovac Biotech's ….* Sinovac-Covid-19	• *Zydus Cadila 's…* Zycovid-D®

* Till August 2021 ; Pharmaceuticals in parantheses are indian partners/ suppliers of global vaccines

Table 26.2 presents salient comparative features of these seven vaccines approved in India However, only three of them – Covishield®, Covaxin® and SputunikV® have been actually used/marketed in India till now being discussed in this chapter. For information about other approved vaccines, see FAQ section.

In addition, over 200 vaccine candidates against Covid-19 are under development, including over 50 in the stage of human trials. Technologically, at least nine different platforms are being used to develop covid vaccines, including *mRNA vaccines* (Comirnaty®, Spikevax®), *DNA vaccines* (ZyCoV-D), Virus vector vaccines (Covishield®, Vaxizevria®, Sputnik V®, Janssen®), Inactivated vaccines (Covaxin®, Coronovac®, Sinopharm® BBIBP-CorV®) and subunit vaccines (Covavax®, Corbevax®).

Contents & Storage : *Covishield®*, also referred as ChAdOx1 nCoV-19 Vaccine, is a recombinant vector vaccine which uses non-replicating chimpanzee adenovirus vector as a shell to envelop the DNA that encodes SARSCoV2 spike glycoprotein propagated in genetically modified human embryonic kidney (HEK) 293 cells. Each dose contains 5×10^{10} viral particles (vp).

Sputnik V® is also a viral vector vaccine, though it uses two different vectors for two doses – rAd26 adenovirus for the first dose and rAd5 adenovirus for the second dose.

Covaxin® is an inactivated whole virion vaccine propagated on a Vero cell-based platform and expressing the viral spike protein of SARS-CoV. Each dose contains 6 µg of Antigen.

All three vaccines need to be stored at 2-8°C and once opened, should only be used within 6 hours or till the end of immunization session, whichever is earlier.

Table 26.2: Comparative information of Common Covid-19 vaccines

	SII	Bharat Biotech	Gamaleya	Zydus-Cadila	Moderna	Astrazeneca	Johnson & Johnson
Brand	Covishield®	Covaxin®	Sputnik V®	Zycov-D	Spikevax®	Vaxzevria®	Janssen®
Type*	vector-based	Inactivated	vector-based	DNA	mRNA	vector-based	vector-based
WHO	Approved	-	-	-	Approved	Approved	Approved
Age limit**	18 yr	18 yr	18 yr	**12 yr**	18 yr	18 yr	18 yr
Doses	2	2	2	**3**	2	2	**1**
Dose interval	12-16 wks	4-8 wks	3 wks	28 days	4 wks	4-12 wks	-
Efficacy	70.42%	77.8%	91.6%	66.6%	94.1%	76%	72%
Efficacy (Severe disease)	-	93.4%.	100%	–	100%	100%	85.9%
Efficacy (Delta variant)	-	65.2%	-	–	-	60%	-
Safety Concerns	Blood clots	-	-	–	Myocarditis Pericarditis[2]	Blood clots	GBS Blood clots
Storage	2-8°C	2-8°C	36-46° F	2-8°C	2-8°C (1 mo)	2-8°C (6+ mo)	36-46°F (3 mo)

*Adenovirus as vector, Sputnik V uses different adenoviruses for two doses. ** Approved lower age limit

Dosage & administration: All three vaccines are given as 0.5 ml/dose intramuscularly over the deltoid region.

Immunization Schedule: All three vaccines are approved for use only at or above 18 years of age, with two doses at a recommended interval of 12-16 weeks for Covishield®, 4-8 weeks for Covaxin® and ≥ 3 weeks for Sputnik V®.

Immunogenicity & protective Efficacy: Correlates of protection are not well established for Covid-19 vaccines, though ≥4-fold rise in S-binding antibodies is generally considered as an indicator of seroconversion,

Covishield® has demonstrated a seroconversion rate of >99% after 28 days second dose with protective efficacy of 70.42% after 14 days of second dose (at 4 week interval). Protective efficacy is higher with increasing dose interval, being 78.79% after two doses at 12 weeks interval. Recent data from UK suggests that AstraZeneca vaccine (similar to Covishield) is also effective against Delta variant (B1.617.2) with ~64% efficacy.

Covaxin®, has been reported to have 77.8% efficacy against symptomatic infections and 93.4% against severe covid disease. Against asymptomatic COVID-19, the efficacy is less i.e. 63.6%. Vaccine also confers 65.2% protection against symptomatic infection with the Delta variant, two weeks after the second dose.

Sputnik V® is 91.6% effective at preventing symptomatic COVID-19 infection and 100% effective at preventing severe infection.

Safety: All three vaccines are safe, though associated with mild to moderate local reactions or systemic side effects e.g.

fever, Chills, headache, myalgia, nausea, fatigue, malaise etc. in ~ 20-50% cases lasting for few days. Adverse reactions are less common and milder after second dose than the first dose. Rare events of Thrombotic-thrombocytopenic events, usually in second week after vaccination, have been reported following Vaxizevria® (AstraZeneca), though a causal relationship has not been established.

Contraindications: All three vaccines are contraindicated in persons with severe allergic reactions e.g. anaphylaxis to the first dose of vaccine. Covid vaccines should also be deferred for - a) Three months after recovery from confirmed Covid disease, b) Two weeks after suspected acute respiratory illness.

Frequently Asked Questions (FAQs)

1. **What is Emergency Use listing (EUL or Emergency use authorization (EUA)?**

    EUL is a risk-based procedure adopted by the WHO to assess and list unlicensed vaccines, therapeutics and *in vitro* diagnostics, in order to expedite availability of these products during a public health emergency. Following criteria must be met by EUL:

    - The disease is serious or immediately life-threatening, with potential to cause an outbreak, epidemic or pandemic;

    - Existing products have not been successful to eradicate the disease or prevent outbreaks;

    - The product is manufactured in compliance with Good Manufacturing Practices (GMP)

    - The applicant undertakes to complete the development of the product and apply for WHO pre-qualification once the product is licensed

In should be noted that EUA does not compromise on safety data and issued only after careful scrutiny of laboratory and clinical trial data, including that on quality, safety, production of protective antibodies and efficacy, followed by a risk-versus- benefit assessment. For COVID-19 vaccines, it has set the bar for minimum efficacy at 50%. Full licensure is obtained when the manufacturer submits the complete data. EUA by Indian regulators is aligned with global guidelines.

2. **What is dubbed as Indian strain or delta strain?**

So called *"Indian strain"* is a double mutant variant of SARS-CoV-2 (B.1.617) with two prominent mutations on positions 452 and 484 of the spike protein. It was actually first sequenced in a global database of COVID-19 variants in October 2020, but went largely unnoticed. The B.1.617 strain carries features from two lineages, the California variants (B.1.427 and B.1.429) and the ones in South Africa (B.1.351) and Brazil (P.1). Widely prevalent in (but not limited to) India, it is believed to be ~60% more contagious than the Alpha variants.

3. **What is a vector in the vector-based vaccines, in context of Covid-19 vaccines?**

Vectors are vehicles which can induce a genetic material from another virus into a cell. Almost all vector-based Covid-19 vaccines use a common-cold Adenovirus as vector, in which the disease causing gene of the virus is replaced by a gene to code the spike (S) proteins and elicit the immune response.

All Oxford-AstraZeneca vaccines (Covishield®, Vaxizevria®, SK bio) as well as Gamalaya's Sputnik V®, and Johnson & Johnson's Janssen® are virus-vector vaccines.

Of these, Sputnik V® uses two different vectors for two different doses, unlike others which use same vector for both doses. (*see main text)

4. **What are mRNA vaccines?**

Conventional vaccines contain live, inactivated or subunit component of a pathogen to trigger the immune response. Unlike these, messenger RNA (mRNA) vaccines are new technology vaccines which do not contain any component of the pathogen but only a genetic code, termed as mRNA. This mRNA is protected by lipid nanoparticles, which also helps its absorption by the cell. When introduced in body, this code instructs host cells to make a piece of corona virus spike protein themselves and express it on the surface to trigger the immune response. These artificially created spike proteins cannot replicate like the original virus. Presently, two marketed vaccines by Pfizer-BioNTech (Comirnaty®) and Moderna (Spikevax®) vaccines have been developed through mRNA technology.

Pfizer- BioNTech's vaccine was the first vaccine to receive WHO-EUL (for use above 12 years) as well as full approval (for use above 16 years), given as two doses at 3-6 weeks interval with 95% efficacy (100% in the age group of 12-15 years). There have been rare reports of myocarditis or pericarditis following this vaccine, though causal association is uncertain.

Moderna's *mRNA1273* vaccine is another mRNA vaccine with 94.1% efficacy (100% for severe disease) licensed for use above 18 years of age (not in 12-18 years age, unlike Pfizer's vaccine) with two doses at 4 weeks interval. With this vaccine too, there have been rare reports of Myocarditis or pericarditis following this vaccine with uncertain causal association.

5. Whether there is a single dose vaccine approved by the WHO against Covid-19?

Johnson & Johnson's Janessen® is a single dose vaccine, approved by the WHO as well as in India. It is an adenoviral vector vaccine to be given as 0.5 ml intramuscularly in persons > 18 years of age (12-17 years under trial) with reported efficacy of 72%-76% against symptomatic disease and 85.9% against severe disease. Vaccine can be stored at 2-8°C for several months. Vaccine is safe except rare events of Thrombotic-thrombocytopenic events, like other virus vector vaccines, without definite causal association.

Convidencia® (AD5-nCOV) is another single dose vaccine developed by Cansino Biologics with 65.7% efficacy against moderate disease and 91% against severe disease. It is not yet launched in India.

6. What are the unique features of ZyCov-D vaccine?

Unique features of Zycov-D vaccine include:

- ZyCov-D® is the first "DNA vaccine" approved for clinical use, using a genetically engineered, non-replicating version of the DNA molecule (plasmid), coded with the instructions to make the spike protein of SARS-CoV-2.

- It is a fully indigenous vaccine, developed with the support of the Department of Biotechnology and the Indian Council of Medical Research and being manufactured by the Zydus Cadila.

- Unlike others, it is a three dose vaccine given at an interval of 28 days between them, using a jet injector, rather than the needle. This injector uses a narrow stream of the fluid to penetrate the skin and deliver the vaccine.

- It is the first vaccine, approved for use in Indian children above 12 years of age with overall reported efficacy of 66%.

7. Which other Covid-19 vaccines are likely to be launched in India in near future?

All WHO approved vaccines are likely to be available soon in India (? except Chinese vaccines BBIBP-CorV® and coronovac®). In addition, two more vaccines are likely to be launched soon in India i.e. Covavax® (Serum institute of India) and Corbevax® (Biological E Limited).

Covavax® is the Indian version of Novavax's NVX-CoV2373 vaccine, which is a protein-subunit vaccine, containing the S-protein of the virus as a nanoparticle to trigger the immune response along with an adjuvant. This vaccine is given as two doses of 0.5 ml intramuscularly at 3 weeks interval with reported efficacy of 90% against symptomatic disease and 100% against the severe disease. Vaccine has very few side effects, though local reactions are more likely due to presence of an adjuvant.

Corbevax is another recombinant protein subunit vaccine, developed by Baylor College of medicine and being manufactured in India by Biological E Limited, which is expected to be available soon.

8. Whether a fully vaccinated person is eligible to travel internationally?

As of now, most countries except some in European Union, recognize travelers with completed doses of any WHO approved vaccine as "Fully immunized", permitted to enter the country. However, Some European countries recognize only those who have received vaccine approved by the European medical agency. Travelers who have received other non-approved vaccines are at a disadvantage as they may not be granted entry to certain countries. In India, Covaxin® and Sputnik V® are not yet approved by WHO, though expected to receive it soon.

8. **Which Covid-19 vaccines are available for use in children, or When?**

As on now, only two Covid vaccines are approved for use in children in 12-18 years age group - *Pfizer-BioNTech's BNT162b2* by the WHO and *Zydus cadila's ZyCov-D* by the India. No vaccine is yet approved for use below 12 years of age, though clinical trials in younger children as young as 6 months are ongoing and vaccines might be available for them by late 2021 or early 2022.

9. **Whether Covid-19 vaccines can be given to Pregnant and lactating mothers?**

Despite the limited data on this vulnerable age group, Government of India has permitted and encouraging the vaccination of all pregnant and lactating mothers due to higher risk of morbidity due to Covid-19 infection in them.

10. **Whether a person with suspected or confirmed Covid infection may be vaccinated?**

All persons, with or without Covid infection in the past need vaccination as the immune response after natural infection is unpredictable. However, those confirmed Covid infection must wait for 3 months before the first dose of vaccine (irrespective of receiving Plasma products). Persons with suspected covid infection must wait for 14 days after recovery to ensure that the infection does not spread from vaccination sites.

References

1. World Health Organization. Covid-19 vaccines: Available at: *https://www.who.int/emergencies/diseases/novel-coronavirus-2019/covid-19-vaccines* (accessed on 24th August 2021).

2. World Health Organization. Covid-19 Vaccine tracker and landscape (Updated till Aug 3rd 2021). Available at: *https://www.who.int/publications/m/item/draft-landscape-of-covid-19-candidate-vaccines* (accessed on 24th August 2021).

3. Center for disease control. Different Covid vaccines (Updated may 27th 2021). Available at *https://www.cdc.gov/coronavirus/2019-ncov/vaccines/different-vaccines.html* (accessed on 26th june 2021).

4. Serum Institute of India. Covishield Fact sheet insert. Available at: *https://www.seruminstitute.com/pdf/covishield_fact_sheet.pdf* (accessed on 13th may 2021).

5. Bharat Biotech. Covaxin Fact sheet. Available at: *https://www.bharatbiotech.com/images/covaxin/covaxin-fact-sheet.pdf* (accessed on 13th may 2021).

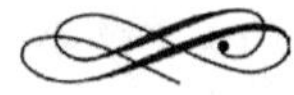

Section

VI

Immunization Under Special Circumstances

Immunocompromized children are in greater need for vaccines due to susceptibility for infections, though benefits may not be optimal in them due to poor or ill-sustained immune response with rapid waning of antibody titers. Moreover, they are also at higher risk of adverse events e.g. development of active disease following live vaccines administration due to uncontrolled replication of the vaccine strains. Efficacy and safety of vaccines in these cases largely depends on severity of the immunosuppression.

General principles for immunization in immunocompromized hosts are as follows, while cause-specific guidelines are discussed in following sections.

- All live vaccines are contraindicated in severe immunodeficiency states but may be given in mild or moderate immunodeficiency after risk-benefit assessment. Immunodeficient cases, if received live vaccines inadvertently, should be watched for adverse effects.

- All inactivated vaccines can be given, though the immunogenicity is unreliable and must be checked periodically with antibody titers if possible, to decide the need for booster doses.

- Higher strength doses and/or more number of doses of inactivated vaccines may be given, if indicated e.g. in HBV vaccination.

- Household contacts of immunocompromized persons should also be fully immunized, including with Inactivated influenza vaccine, to reduce the risk of transmission. However, they should not receive transmissible vaccines e.g. OPV (to be replaced with IPV).

- Highly immunocompromized patients should avoid handling diapers of infants who have been vaccinated with RV vaccine for 4 weeks.

- Post-exposure prophylaxis e.g. for rabies or tetanus, needs to be more intensive with lower threshold for passive prophylaxis in these cases.

27.1: HUMAN IMMUNODEFICIENCY VIRUS INFECTION (HIV/AIDS)

Spectrum of Immunosuppression in HIV-infected children spans from Asymptomatic infection to Full-blown AIDS with severe Immunosuppression. Since majority of these children are infected at birth but remain asymptomatic or un-diagnosed at the time of initial immunization visits, decision to vaccinate usually depends on their general clinical status. Some general consideration for immunization in HIV infected children are as follows –

- All vaccines, including the live vaccines, are recommended in asymptomatic children, though Inactivated vaccines are preferable, if possible (e.g. IPV instead of OPV).

- In a symptomatic child, all live vaccines are forbidden, but at times MR/MMR and varicella vaccines may be considered after risk-benefit assessment.

- Since the immunogenicity may be unreliable or wanes early, monitoring of antibody titers is desirable after vaccination and periodically to assess the need of boosters. Other strategies e.g. double dose or additional dose for primary vaccination are also used for selected vaccines e.g. HBV to ensure adequate immune response.

Table 27.1 provides a summary of IAP recommendations for immunization in HIV infected children.

Table 27.1: IAP recommendations for vaccination of HIV-infected children.

Vaccine	Asymptom-atic	Symptomatic
BCG	Yes	No
DPT	Yes	
HIB	Yes	
HBV	Four doses, Double dose, Check for Seroconversion, booster if required	
IPV/OPV	Yes, Preferably IPV, IPV also to contacts	
RV	Yes	No, Insufficient data
PCV	Yes	
PPSV	Two dose at 2 yr age (after 2 mo of PCV) and at 5 yrs of first dose	
Influenza	Yes, use Inactivated vaccine	
MR/MMR	Yes*	No, if CD4 <15%
Varicella	Yes*	No if CD4 >15% < 5 yrs for > 6 mo CD4 count > 200 > 5 yrs for > 6 mo
HAV	yes	Yes, check for Seroconversion, Booster if required.
Typhoid	Yes	
HPV	Yes	
Yellow fever	Yes	No

* After Risk-benefit assessment
Source: NACO guidelines 2018

27.2: CONGENITAL IMMUNODEFICIENCY DISORDERS

Congenital immunodeficiency disorders encompass large number of dieases with variable severity and components of Immunosupppression. Immunization guidelines for Congenital Immunodeficiency disorders differ according to the basic defect and some general principles are as follows –

a) **Severe T cell immunodeficiencies (SCID):** All live vaccines are contraindicated and inactivated vaccines are ineffective. Patients who have received live vaccines e.g. BCG prior to diagnosis have a higher risk of complications e.g. disseminated disease. Risk-specific vaccines i.e. PCV and HIB are recommended though response is variable.

b) **Severe B cell immunodeficiency** (X-linked agamma-globulinemia): Live bacterial vaccines e.g. BCG, OPV and LAIV are contraindicated. Live viral vaccines e.g. MMR and Varicella may be given but are usually ineffective due to concomitant Immunoglobulin therapy. Inactivated vaccines, other than IIV, are not routinely administered to patients during immunoglobulin therapy but may be given as part of immune response assessment prior to starting the therapy. Risk-specific vaccines i.e. PCV and HIB are recommended in these children. In less severe B cell deficiencies e.g. IgA and IgG subclass deficiencies, only OPV is contraindicated.

c) **Combined immunodeficiencies** such as Di George syndrome, Wiskott-Aldrich syndrome and ataxia telangiectasia. Inactivated vaccines may be given but live vaccines are contraindicated.

d) **Complement deficiencies:** All vaccines can be safely given with no contraindications. These children are at higher risk for infections due to capsulated organisms and must receive all age-appropriate immunizations with special reference to PCV/PPSV, MCV and Hib vaccines.

e) **Phagocyte defects:** Live bacterial vaccines e.g. BCG, are contraindicated in phagocytic defects but all inactivated vaccines are safe and likely to be effective. Live viral vaccines e.g. MMR and varicella are contraindicated in phagocyte defects which are undefined or have associated T cell and natural killer (NK) cell dysfunction e.g. Chediak-Higashi syndrome, Leukocyte adhesion deficiency, Myeloperoxidase deficiency etc. PCV/PPSV vaccines are specifically recommended.

27.3: CANCERS AND CHEMOTHERAPY

Cancer cases, specially those on chemotherapy, are at higher risk of infections including those by vaccine-preventable diseases. However, vaccine uptake is unreliable during and for some time even after stoppage of chemotherapy. Pre-existing immunity also wanes due to the disease and chemotherapy and needs boosting on Recovery.

Severity of the immunosuppression in cancers varies from minimal in solid tumors to extensive in hematological malignancies, Some malignancies e.g. Lymphoma present with specific immune involvement e.g. lack of lymphocytic response to various antigens.

In general, Influence of cancer *per se* on immune functions is minimal, largely caused by chemotherapy and to a lesser extent, by radiotherapy. Degree of chemotherapy-induced immunosuppression depends on the intensity, duration and nature of component drugs. Both cellular and humoral immunity are affected due to involvement of the T-cell/ Natural killer (NK) cells and B-lymphocytes respectively.

Highly immunocompromized cancer patients include those with – a) generalized or hematological malignancy, b) chemo/ radiotherapy in preceding three months, c) steroid therapy > 20 mg prednisolone equivalent daily for > 2 weeks, and d) stem cell transplant within preceding 2 years or with ongoing evidence of Graft *versus* Host disease (GVHD).

Some general considerations for immunization of cancer patients, according to IAP recommendations 2019[3], are as follows –

- *No vaccine is recommended during chemotherapy including Pulse polio doses, and for next 6 month after stoppage of treatment, except Influenza and HBV.*

- IIV is recommended to all children during chemotherapy with single dose annually before the peak season (Two doses at one month interval in those below 9 years, if not received earlier) However, Influenza vaccine beyond one year of completion of chemotherapy is not recommended unless child continues to have other high-risk conditions.

- HBV vaccine is recommended during chemotherapy *only* in previously unimmunized children with four doses at 0, 1, 2 and 12 months in double the usual doses along with age appropriate dose of HBIG every three months, till no risk of blood product exposure.

- IIV and varicella vaccines are also recommended to the siblings and parents while OPV is contraindicated in siblings (to be replaced by IPV, if needed) including pulse polio doses. If OPV is administered to a sibling by mistake, s/he should remain away from index child for at least 2 weeks.

- Post-exposure prophylaxis for rabies during chemotherapy must include - a) Passive prophylaxis with RBIG/ Monoclonal antibodies even for Category-II bites and b) Six doses of ARV, including the 6th dose on day 90.

- Tetanus prophylaxis in wound management during chemotherapy must include - a) single TT booster dose in all cases irrespective of previous immunization status, and b) TIG, except in cases with clean and minor wounds.

- Post-exposure varicella prophylaxis is recommended during chemotherapy with VZIG, IVIG or High dose Acyclovir in exposed children, preferably after assessing varicella-IgG levels before prophylaxis. (*IM-VZIG* 250 mg (< 5 yrs); 500 mg (5-10 yr); 750 mg (11-14 yr) or 1000 mg (>15 yrs) or *IVIG* as 0.2 gm/kg or *PO Ayclovir* from day 7 to day 21 of exposure as 200 mg QID < 2 yrs; 400 mg QID for 2-6 yrs: 800 mg QID > 6 yrs).

- Post-chemotherapy, immunization depends on the previous immunization status and should begin only after 6 months of completion of chemotherapy. While unimmunized or partially immunized children should receive catch-up immunization as per usual recommendations, fully immunized children before chemotherapy should receive *a single booster dose of age appropriate DPT, IPV, HBV, HIB, PCV,HAV, TCV, MMR and Varicella.* In children, who had received only OPV doses during previous immunization, two IPV doses at one month interval are recommended. Data is insufficient to recommend HPV Booster, though may be considered in females.

27.4: CORTICOSTEROIDS OR OTHER IMMUNOSUPPRESSIVE THERAPY

Efficacy of inactivated vaccines as well as safety and efficacy of live vaccines is doubtful in cases on prolonged corticosteroid therapy and general considerations for immunization in them are as follows –

- Children on low-dose systemic steroids or topical or inhaled steroids may be safely and effectively immunized with all vaccines.

- Children on high-dose oral corticosteroids (Prednisolone > 2 mg/kg/day or 20 mg/day or equivalent) for >2 weeks should not receive live virus vaccines until steroids have been discontinued for at least one month.

- Children with other immunosuppressant medications e.g. biologic immune modulators e.g. Rituximab or TNF-α, should also not receive live virus vaccines during therapy, except in special circumstances.

27.5: HEMATOPOIETIC STEM CELL TRANSPLANTS (HSCT)

HSCT Recipients are virtually unimmunized due to loss of all memory responses during marrow ablation and need to be re-immunized. At the same time they are immunocompromized with higher risk of infections as well as unreliable efficacy and safety of vaccines.

Some basic considerations in immunizations of HSCT cases (**Table 27.2**)[2] are as follows –

- It is advisable to complete age-appropriate immunization of the donor as his/her vaccination has been shown to improve post-transplant immunity in recipients. However, safety of live vaccines in the donor within preceding 4 weeks of stem-cell harvesting is uncertain and should be avoided.

- It is advisable to complete age-appropriate immunization, including PCV/PPSV, in Recipients at least 4 weeks before the conditioning period for live vaccines and 2 weeks before the inactivated vaccines. Although these recipients lose all immune responses during conditioning, it is likely that some protection may persist.

- Post-HSCT, recipients should be considered as *"never vaccinated"* regardless of pre-HSCT vaccination status and they need to be *re-immunized* with all age-appropriate inactivated vaccines, after 6 months of procedure. Heavy immunosuppression in early Post-HSCT phase necessitates a minimum time gap of 6 months before initiation of re-immunization. However, some vaccines e.g. PCV and IIV can be given after 3-4 months (**Table 27.2**).

- Additional doses may be needed for HBV (if seroconversion is not achieved) or PCV13 (4th dose in cases of chronic GVHD).

- Live vaccines should not be administered to HSCT patients with active GVHD or ongoing immunosuppression. MMR and varicella vaccines may be administered after 24 months, if the recipient is presumed to be immunocompetent and 8-11 months after last dose of IVIG.

27.6: SOLID ORGAN TRANSPLANTS (SOT)

SOT recipients are immunocompromized even before the transplant due to the underlying disease and continue to be the same after procedure due to immunosuppressive therapy or Graft rejection.

Some important considerations related to immunization for solid organ transplant recipients (**Table 27.2**)[2] are as follows -

- SOT Recipients should complete all age-appropriate immunizations, including PCV/PPSV, prior to the transplant, preferably in early disease, when they are less immunosuppressed.

- Pre-transplant immunization may be provided with accelerated schedule if required and must be completed at least 4 weeks before the procedure, specially for live vaccines. Seroconversion should be documented before transplant, if possible. In these cases, Varicella and MMR vaccines may be given even at 6-11 months of age.

- Post-transplant immunization in SOT aims to complete catch-up immunization. Optimal time to begin vaccines after the procedure is uncertain, though inactivated vaccines can be given after 6 months, when immunosuppression has been reduced. It is desirable to check antibody titers (HAV, HBV) after 6 months of transplant, to decide the need for boosters.

- IIV can be given even in immediate transplant period despite intensive immunosuppression.

- All live vaccines are contraindicated after the transplant. However household and health-care contacts of SOT recipients should be immunized with live vaccines e.g. MMR, Varicella etc and influenza to reduce the risk of transmission.

Table 27.2: Post-Transplant Immunization recommendations

Vaccine	HSCT		SOT	
	Post-Transplant (Re-Immunization)	Time-Gap	Post-Transplant (Catch-up immunization)	Time-Gap
DPT	< 7 yr: DTaP (0, 1, 6 mo) > 7 yr: Tdap>Td>Td (0, 1, 6 mo)	6 mo	If not completed earlier	6 mo
IPV	0,1,6 mo	3 mo	If not completed earlier	6 mo
HBV	0,1,6 mo	6 mo	If not completed earlier	6 mo
Hib	0,1,6 mo	3 mo	If not completed earlier	6 mo
HAV	0, 6 mo	6 mo	If not completed earlier	6 mo
PCV13	0,1, 2 mo	3 mo	If not completed earlier	6 mo
PPSV23	Single dose, if no GVHD	12 mo	If not completed earlier	6 mo
Influenza	Two doses in first year at 0, 1 mo then Single dose annually	4 mo	Single dose annually	Soon after transplant
MCV	0 and 3 mo	6 mo	If not completed earlier	6 mo
RV	Contraindicated	-	Contraindicated	-
Varicella	Contraindicated*	-	Contraindicated	-
MMR	Contraindicated*	-	Contraindicated	-

* MMR and Varicella vaccines may be given after 24 months if recipients is presumed to be immunocompetent, (8-11months after last dose of IVIG).

27.7: SPLENIC DYSFUNCTION (ASPLENIA, SPLENICTOMY, SICKLE CELL DISEASE)

Splenic functions are compromised in cases of congenital Asplenia or hyposplenia or secondary to Sickle cell disease, Splenectomy or radiation therapy. These children are at high risk of serious infections with encapsulated organisms. Some important immunization considerations in these cases are as follows –

a) No vaccine, including live vaccines, is contraindicated and they should receive all age-appropriate regular vaccines, with special emphasis on PCV, HIB, and Typhoid vaccines.

b) In addition, they should also receive – a) Two doses of MCV at 8 weeks interval after 2 years of age; b) Single dose of HIB vaccine, if not received till 5 years of age, c) Age-appropriate dose/s of PCV, and d) A single dose of PPSV, repeated once after 5 years. (A minimum gap of 8 weeks should be maintained between PCV and PPSV).

c) *For planned Splenectomy*, PPSV should be given at least 2 weeks prior to surgery. Children who have received PPSV earlier but not the PCV, should also receive recommended PCV dose at least 8 weeks after PPSV.

d) *For emergency Splenectomy*, vaccination should begin at least 2 weeks after the surgery rather than immediately, for better antibody response with - a) MCV-Dose 1, PCV and HIB (if not received earlier), followed after 8 week by – b) MCV-Dose 2 and PPSV23. PPSV23 must be repeated once after 5 years.

27.8: ANATOMIC BARRIERS DEFECTS: COCHLEAR IMPLANTS, CSF LEAKS ETC

These children should receive all age-appropriate immunizations, with special reference to PCV as per recommended schedule, followed by PPSV23 after 8 weeks and minimum 2 weeks before cochlear implant surgery.

Frequently Asked Questions (FAQs)

1. **Whether a baby born to HIV-infected mother may be given BCG and OPV before discharge from nursery?**

   All HIV-exposed infants should be given BCG at birth, as they are unlikely to be immunocompromized at birth, even if infected. However Birth dose of OPV may be avoided in an individual case, due to potential risk of infection to immunocompromized mother due to shedding of the virus in stools of the newborn.

2. **Whether Rotavirus vaccines may be given to an HIV-exposed infant?**

   Rotavirus vaccine is recommended to all HIV-exposed infants as they are - a) more vulnerable to diarrhea, and b) Unlikely to have confirmed diagnosis or severe immunodeficiency. However, mothers, if significantly immunocompromized, should avoid handling of their diapers for 4 weeks, as virus is excreted in stools.

3. **How can we improve protective efficacy of inactivated vaccines in a immunocompromized child?**

   Immunogenicity of inactivated vaccines is unreliable in immunocompromized children and hence – a) Antibody titers must be checked periodically, if possible, to determine the need for booster doses, and b) Additional doses or Double-dose vaccines may be given, if indicated e.g. in HBV vaccination.

4. **Which vaccines are contraindicated in siblings of a immunocompromized child.**

   Household contacts e.g. siblings of immunocompromized persons should not receive transmissible vaccines e.g. OPV, which may be replaced with IPV. If administered tby chance, s/he should remain away from index child for at least 2 weeks.

5. **Whether Pulse polio vaccine can be given to a immuno-compromized child?**

    Pulse polio immunization should be avoided in HIV-infected child, specially if symptomatic, due to – a) inherent risk of a live OPV vaccine e.g. VDPV; and b) potential risk of infection to immunocompromized mother due to shedding of the virus in stools of vaccinated infant.

6. **Whether Pulse polio vaccine may be given to a child on chemotherapy?**

    No vaccine is recommended during chemotherapy including Pulse polio doses, and for next 6 month after stoppage of treatment, except Influenza and HBV.

7. **A child on chemotherapy was bitten by a dog? What is the difference in post-exposure prophylaxis for this child vs a healthy child.**

    Post-exposure prophylaxis for rabies during chemotherapy must include - a) Passive prophylaxis with RBIG/Monoclonal antibodies even for Category-II bites and b) Six doses of ARV, including the 6th dose on day 90.

8. **A child on chemotherapy sustained wounds during a vehicular accident. What is the difference in post-exposure prophylaxis for this child *vis a vis* a healthy child?**

    Tetanus prophylaxis in wound management during chemotherapy must include - a) single TT booster dose in all cases irrespective of previous immunization status, and b) TIG in all cases, except those with clean and minor wounds.

9. **Whether a child on MDI steroids can receive live vaccines?**

    Children on low-dose systemic steroids or topical or inhaled steroids may be safely and effectively immunized with all vaccines.

10. **How long should one wait to being Immunizations after chemotherapy and transplants?**

A six month interval is generally recommended before resuming immunizations in a child on chemotherapy or stem-cell/solid-organ transplant, with some exceptions (see Table 27.2).

11. **A child on chemotherapy for lymphoma was fully vaccinated for his age before the diagnosis. Whether he needs any further vaccinations?**

In addition to further age-appropriate doses, all fully immunized children before the chemotherapy should receive *a single booster dose of DPT/Tdap, IPV, HBV, HIB, PCV,HAV, Typhoid, MMR and Varicella.* Those who had received only OPV doses earlier, must also be given two doses of IPV at one month interval. Data is insufficient to recommend HPV Booster, though may be considered in females.

12. **A 2 year old boy with Nephrotic syndrome on treatment was not vaccinated beyond 10 weeks of age. Whether and when he can resume vaccination?**

Children on high-dose oral corticosteroids (Prednisolone > 2 mg/kg/day or 20 mg/day or equivalent) for > 2 weeks should not receive live virus vaccines until steroids have been discontinued for at least one month.

13. **Why do we need to revaccinate all children after HSCT?**

HSCT Recipients lose all memory responses during conditioning i.e. marrow ablation. Post-HSCT, they should be considered as "never vaccinated" regardless of pre-HSCT status and need to be *re-immunized* with all age-appropriate inactivated vaccines, after 6 months of procedure with some exceptions (see Table 27.2).

14. **Which vaccines should be received by prospective kidney transplant patients before the surgery?**

Prospective SOT Recipients should complete all age-appropriate immunizations, including PCV/PPSV at least 4 weeks before surgery, preferably in the early stage of primary disease, when they are less immunosuppressed. If required, some vaccines e.g. Varicella and MMR vaccines may be given even before the recommended age i.e. 6-11 months.

15. **Which vaccines are advisable to health care professionals working in a Transplant unit?**

Health-care workers as well as household contacts of SOT recipients should be immunized up-to-date with live vaccines e.g. MMR, Varicella etc and influenza vaccine to reduce the risk of transmission.

16. **A 6 year old child has undergone emergency splenectomy after vehicular accident 7 days back. Which vaccines he needs now on priority basis and when?**

In this case, vaccination should begin at least 2 weeks after the surgery rather than immediately, for better antibody response with - a) MCV-Dose 1, PCV and HIB (if not received earlier), followed after 8 week by – b) MCV-Dose 2 and PPSV23. PPSV23 must be repeated once after 5 years. In addition, he should also receive age-appropriate catch-up immunization in due course.

17. **Which vaccines are recommended for a child planned for cochlear implant after 2 months?**

Children undergoing cochlear implant surgery are at risk for meningitis and must receive – a)Two doses of MCV at 8 weeks interval after 2 years of age; b) Single dose of HIB vaccine, if not received earlier till 5 years of age, c) age-appropriate dose/s of PCV, if not received earlier, and

d) Single dose of PPSV, repeated once after 5 years. (A minimum gap of 8 weeks should be maintained between PCV and PPSV).

References

1. Rubin GL, Levin MJ, Ljungman P, et al. 2013 IDSA clinical practice guidelines for vaccination of the immunocompromized host. Clin Infect Dis. 2014;58:e44-100.
2. L'Hullier AG, Kumar D. Immunizations in solid organ and hematopoietic stem cell transplant patients: A comprehensive review. Hum Vaccin Immunother. 2015;11:2852-63.
3. Moulik NR et al. Immunization of Children with Cancer in India Treated with Chemotherapy – Consensus Guideline from the Pediatric Hematology-Oncology Chapter and the Advisory Committee on Vaccination and Immunization Practices of the Indian Academy of Pediatrics. Ind Pediatr 2019; 56:1041-1048.
4. National AIDS control organization: Assessment of Children with HIV Infection, Pre-ART Care and Follow Up. *In:* National Technical Guidelines on antiretroviral treatment. October 2018. Available at - *https://lms.naco.gov.in/ frontend/content/NACO%20-%20National%20Technical%20Guidelines%20on%20 ART_October%202018%20(1).pdf.* (Accessed on 16th may.2021).
5. Shastri D. Immunization in Special situations. *In:* IAP Guidebook on Immunization 2018-19 - Advisory Committee on Vaccines and Immunization Practices, Indian Academy of Pediatrics, 3[r]d Edition, New Delhi, Jaypee Brothers 2020; pp 404-432.
6. Mitra M. Vaccination in special situations. *In:* Vashishtha V et al. FAQs on Vaccines and immunization practices. 2nd Edition. .New Delhi, Jaypee Brothers 2015; pp 54-62.
7. American Academy of Pediatrics. Immunization in special circumstances. Red Book® 2021-2024 Report of the Committee on Infectious Diseases. Kimberlin Et al (Eds), 32nd Edition, 2021; pg 67-99.

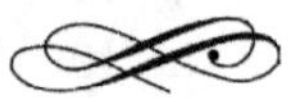

Children with health issues other than immunocompromized states (Chapter 27) or on some medications may also need modifications in their immunization schedule, as discussed in this section.

28.1: PRETERM / LOW BIRTH WEIGHT INFANTS

Three major issues related to immunizations of preterm and LBW infants are high risk of infections and other medical problems, uncertain immunogenicity due to physiologically immature immune system and logistic problems to given vaccines to a very small child.

Some basic considerations regarding immunization of these children are as follows -

- BCG and OPV may be administered at birth irrespective of the weight or gestational age, after stabilization and before discharge. However, HBV birth dose should be delayed till one month of age in babies weighing less than 2000 gms at birth due to doubtful immunogenicity in them, *unless* delivered to an HBsAg positive mother.

- All subsequent vaccines may be given as per chronologic age (even if still in hospital), except RV vaccine, which should be deferred until discharge to prevent the health care-associated spread of virus in nursery.

- Since preterm and low birth weight babies have low muscle mass, smaller and thinner needles must be used in them for intramuscular injections.

- PCV, RV and Influenza vaccines are highly recommended in these children, due to their increased susceptibility to infections.

- It is advisable to ascertain appropriate immunizations of health care personnel and household contacts handing these babies to minimize the risk of transmission.

28.2: ACUTE OR CHRONIC DISEASES

Infections and illnesses are common in children during immunization visits, necessitating decision-making to continue, defer, modify or refuse immunizations for the time being or all together. Some general considerations for immunization in sick children at the time of immunization visit are as follows –

a) Vaccinations can be safely given during *minor illnesses* like upper respiratory tract infections, mild diarrhea, and otitis media.

b) Vaccination may be postponed during *moderate or severe acute illness* to avoid superimposing vaccine reaction (e.g. Febrile seizures), which may be wrongly attributed to the vaccine, posing medico-legal issues and discrediting the vaccine. However, parents should be instructed to visit again, as soon as the child is better, for postponed vaccine dose.

c) No vaccine is contraindicated in children with *chronic systemic diseases*. In fact, these cases might be more susceptible for specific infections and need special vaccines depending on the type of disease e.g. HBV in chronic liver disease, Pneumococcal and influenza vaccines in cardiopulmonary disease etc.

Immunogenicity and duration of protection of vaccines

may be unreliable in children with chronic illnesses and need periodic assessment of antibody response, with boosters, if necessary. Immunization with higher antigen content or more doses of vaccines (e.g. HBV) may be useful in these cases.

d) Children with *hemorrhagic disorders or on anticoagulants* are at risk for bleeding following intramuscular injections. In these cases, some vaccines can be given subcutaneously, if equally immunogenic e.g. IPV, PPV and Hib. Essentially Intramuscular vaccines can be given with a thinner needle and applying the firm pressure without rubbing over injection site for 5-10 minutes. In severe cases, vaccination may be given shortly after administration of clotting-factor.

28.3: HISTORY OF ALLERGY

Hypersensitivity reactions to vaccines may be due to the active antigen *per se*, or more likely due to other additives in finished product e.g. preservatives, stabilizers or even diluents. Most of these reactions are mild and self-limiting e.g. urticaria, though life-threatening anaphylaxis is rare but major concern in these cases. Some general considerations for immunization in children with history of allergy are as follows –

a) Hypersensitivity reactions are unpredictable and all vaccinees should be observed for at least 15-30 minutes after vaccination, with resuscitation facility in standby.

b) Atopic children and those with family history of atopy are not at higher risk for allergic reactions following vaccinations, though should be monitored carefully.

c) Children with history of serious egg allergy should avoid vaccines containing residual proteins e.g. Yellow fever and Q-fever. Other vaccines of concern in them are Influenza, Varicella, MMR and some Rabies vaccines, due to use of chick-embryo cultures in the manufacturing process. However, the amount of residual protein (Ovalbumin) in modern vaccines is too low to elicit severe allergic reactions and *Egg allergy is not a contraindication for Influenza, Varicella or MMR vaccinations.*

d) Neomycin, Gelatin and Latex (used in vial-lids or applicators) are other common causes of vaccine allergy and children with known history of serious hypersensitivity or anaphylaxis to any such vaccine components should not be given these vaccines..

e) A mild hypersensitivity reaction to the previous dose is not a contraindication to further doses of same vaccine, though the child should be observed for a longer time and resuscitation equipment should be kept standby.

f) A serious hypersensitivity reaction e.g. anaphylaxis to the previous dose is the absolute contraindication for the same or related vaccines e.g. DTaP and MMR is also contraindicated after anaphylaxis to DTwP and MR vaccination respectively. However, other vaccines may be given.

28.4: CONCOMITANT ANTIMICROBIAL THERAPY

All vaccines can be given during antimicrobial therapy with no effect on immune responses barring few exceptions –

a) Live influenza vaccine should not be given to a child on antiviral drugs e.g. Oseltamivir, until 48 hours of cessation of therapy, though these drugs have no effect on immune responses to inactivated Influenza vaccines.

b) Antiviral drugs against herpesviruses (e.g., acyclovir or valacyclovir) might reduce the efficacy of live attenuated varicella vaccines and should be discontinued at least 24 hours before vaccination, if possible.

c) Concomitant INH administration might affect uptake of live attenuated BCG vaccine, though not significantly and INH prophylaxis is not a contraindication for BCG vaccination at birth.

28.5. BLOOD PRODUCT INFUSIONS

Blood products (whole blood, packed red blood cells, plasma, and platelets) as well as other antibody-containing blood products (IVIG, IMIG, HBIG, TIG, VZIG, RBIG) may inhibit the immune response to live vaccines for variable period of time, depending on the amount of antigen-specific antibodies present in the product. Some basic considerations for immunization in recipients of blood or antibody products in recent past are as follows –

a) Inactivated, recombinant and polysaccharide vaccines as well as toxoids can be administered simultaneously, before or after an antibody-containing product without any interval criteria, but at different sites, using the standard recommended dose.

b) Live vaccines e.g. Measles and varicella, should not be administered simultaneously or at an interval shorter than recommended with blood/antibody containing products (**Table 28.1**). If unavoidable, the dose should be repeated or antibody titers must be checked after the recommended period. However, in unimmunized contacts with measles exposure during deferment interval, additional doses of IgG or Measles vaccine might be indicated.

c) Other live vaccines e.g. yellow fever, Rotavirus vaccine, live attenuated influenza vaccine, and zoster vaccines

Table 28.1: Recommended time-gap between blood/Antibody products and Live vaccines*

Blood/Antibody product	Time-interval	Antibody product	Time-interval
Whole blood/Packed RBCs	6 mo	Tetanus Ig	3 mo
Plasma, Platelet products	7 mo	Hepatitis B Ig	3 mo
Washed RBCs	None	Hepatitis A Ig	3 mo
RBCs- adenine saline added	3 mo	Rabies Ig	4 mo
IVIG (400 mg/kg)	8 mo	Varicella Ig	4 mo
IVIG (1-2 g/kg)	10/11 mo	CMV- Ig	6 mo
Measles-Ig (40/80 mg/kg)	5/6 mo	Monoclonal RSV-AB	None

* Excluding yellow fever, Rotavirus, live attenuated influenza and zoster vaccines, which can be administered any time, if required.

may be administered at any time before, concurrent with, or after administration of these products.

d) Low dose anti-D globulin given to postpartum Rh-negative women is not an indication to defer Rubella or Varicella vaccination to unimmunized ones, who should be vaccinated immediately after giving birth and, if possible, tested after 3 months to ensure immunity to Rubella and Measles.

e) Administration of an antibody-containing product within 14 days of MR/MMR or Varicella vaccine might affect the vaccine uptake and the dose should be repeated after recommended time interval, unless serologic testing indicates protective antibody titers.

Frequently Asked Questions (FAQs)

1. **Whether a boy with hemophilia can be given routine vaccines?**

   Children with bleeding disorders e.g. hemophilia are at risk of developing bleeding/hematoma at the site of injection and following general principles must be used in them –

   - Vaccines, which can be given subcutaneously or intradermally without compromising the efficacy e.g. HBV, HAV, IPV, PPSV, ARV etc., must be given through these alternative routes.

   - A finer-bore needle (23 G or More) should be used for injections, followed by firm pressure at the site for at least two minutes without rubbing.

   - Injections should preferably be scheduled soon after factor replacement therapy (<12-24 hours), if possible.

   - Parents should be counseled about the risk *versus* benefits of vaccination and potential indicators of bleeding/hematoma to contact the doctor. NSAIDs, other than Paracetamol, must be avoided for pain due to risk of bleeding.

2. **A five-year old fully immunized boy developed Guillain-Barre syndrome 5 days after receiving MMR-3 vaccine and treated with IV Immunoglobulins. What are the implications for vaccination in this case.**

   This child is due to receive DPT, IPV and MMR at this age and –

   - All non-live vaccines e.g. DPT and IPV can be given without any specific time-interval.

   - MMR-3 must be repeated after 10-11 months (**Table 28.1**) of IVIG Therapy as an antibody-containing product given within 14 days of administering a live vaccine might have interefered with its uptake, which should not be considered as a valid dose.

3. **Whether a Thalassemic child can be given due vaccines on next day of blood transfusion, before discharge.**

All inactivated vaccines and oral live vaccines can be given just before or after blood transfusion. Live vaccines e.g. Measles or Varicella, can also be given without delay, if washed RBCs were used for transfusions. However, an interval of 6 months is required between whole blood/ Packed cell transfusions and live vaccines.

4. **Whether a child with strong family history of Atopy may be given a vaccine?**

Family history of Atopy is not a contraindication of vaccination, though regular precaution of 15-30 minutes observation after injection with standby resuscitation facility to manage severe allergic reactions must be followed.

5. **Whether a child with egg allergy can be given all vaccines?**

Children with egg allergy should avoid vaccines containing significant amount of residual egg proteins e.g. Yellow fever. Other vaccines of concern are Influenza, Varicella, MMR and some Rabies vaccines (PCEV) due to use of chick-embryo cultures in the manufacturing process. However, the amount of residual protein (Ovalbumin) in these vaccines is too low to elicit severe allergic reactions and egg allergy is not a contraindication for these vaccinations.

6. **Whether a hospitalized child on antibiotics can be immunized for all due vaccines?**

All due vaccines can be given to a stable hospitalized

child unless otherwise contraindicated. Antibiotics do not affect uptake of vaccines. In fact, Hospitalization is an opportunity to complete age-appropriate immunization before discharge. However, vaccines which are excreted in stools e.g. Rotavirus vaccines and OPV (except Pulse Polio doses) should be deferred till discharge to avoid health care-associated spread of virus.

7. **Whether a hospitalized child with suspected influenza on Oseltamivir therapy can be given Influenza vaccine at discharge?**

Antiviral drugs e.g. oseltamivir do not affect immune response to inactivated vaccines and this child can be given IIV, even on oseltamivir therapy. However, Live viral vaccines e.g. Live influenza or Varicella vaccines should be deferred to 48 hours and 24 hours respectively after stopping corresponding antiviral drugs e.g. Osletamivir or Acyclovir.

8. **Which vaccines can be given to a 32 week preterm baby weighing 1.6 kg?**

BCG and OPV must be administered at birth irrespective of the weight or gestational age, after stabilization and before discharge. However, Birth-dose of HBV birth should be delayed till one month of age in babies weighing < 2 Kg due to doubtful immunogenicity, unless delivered to an HBsAg positive mother.

References

1. Centers for Disease Control and Prevention (CDC). General Recommendations on Immunization. Recommendations of the Advisory Committee on Immunization Practices. MMWR. 2019;60:1-61.

2. National Hemophilia Foundation. MASAC Recommendations on administration of vaccines to individuals with bleeding disorders. available at - *https://www.hemophilia.org/healthcare-professionals/guidelines-on-care/masac-*

documents/masac-document-221-recommendations-on-administration-of-vaccines-to-individuals-with-bleeding-disorders (accessed on 6th July 2021).

3. Shastri D. Immunization in Special situations. In: IAP Guidebook on Immunization 2018-19 - Advisory Committee on Vaccines and Immunization Practices, Indian Academy of Pediatrics, 3rd Edition, New Delhi, Jaypee Brothers 2020; pp 404-432.

4. Mitra M. Vaccination in special situations. In: Vashishtha V et al. FAQs on Vaccines and immunization practices. 2nd Edition. New Delhi, Jaypee Brothers 2015; pp 54-62.

5. American Academy of Pediatrics. Immunization in special circumstances. Red Book® 2021-2024 Report of the Committee on Infectious Diseases. Kimberlin Et al (Eds), 32nd Edition, 2021; pg 67-99.

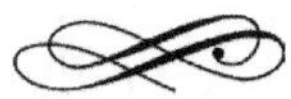

Maternal Immunization

Pregnancy and lactation are vulnerable age groups, with safety and efficacy concerns not only for the vaccinees themselves but also for their offsprings. Important guidelines for immunization in these situations are discussed in this section.

29.1. IMMUNIZATION IN PREGNANCY

Antenatal Immunizations offer an opportunity to protect not only the mother but also her newborn baby through passive transfer of antibodies. However, pregnancy is also a period of physiological immunosuppression with safety issues following live vaccines, including potential risk of transfer of vaccine induced infection to the fetus.

Some general considerations for immunization of pregnant mothers are as follows –

- All pregnant women are recommended Td immunization under NIS, with two doses at 4 weeks interval, starting as early as possible with last dose at least 2 weeks before delivery. Mothers, who had received two doses in previous pregnancy within last 3 years, need only a single booster Td dose.

- IAP recommends to replace first dose of Td with *Tdap* followed by second dose as Td after one month, to reduce the burden of pertussis in young infants till the primary series... Every subsequent pregnancy must receive one Tdap dose, preferably in last trimester.

- Inactivated influenza vaccine is recommended to all pregnant women due to substantial risk of severe disease during pregnancy, potential benefit of preventing disease in young infants due to transplacental transfer of antibodies and established safety record. However, *Live attenuated influenza vaccine should not be used during pregnancy.*

- *Live vaccines e.g. MMR are contraindicated during pregnancy* and conception should be avoided for at least 4 weeks after vaccination. However, routine pregnancy test is not recommended before MMR vaccination and termination of pregnancy is not warranted, if the vaccine has been received inadvertently in this period.

- Yellow fever vaccine should be avoided in pregnancy but may be given if the travel is unavoidable as the risk of infection outweighs the risk of vaccination (preferably in First trimester).

- All inactivated vaccines, including rabies vaccine and immunoglobulins can be safely given during pregnancy, if required.

- All pregnant women should be tested for HbsAg and if positive, should be followed carefully to ensure that their newborns receive due care at birth.

- All pregnant women should be evaluated for Rubella, Varicella, and HBV immunization and if unimmunized, should be vaccinated immediately *after delivery.*

- MR/MMR and varicella vaccines can be safely given to contacts of pregnant women.

- CDC recommends any Covid-19 vaccine to pregnant women as - a) They are at higher risk of Covid-19 related morbidity, and b) No safety concerns have been reported with any licensed vaccines in United states to mother or her baby.

- Federation of Obstetrics and Gynaecology of India (FOGSI) has also recommended Covid-19 vaccines to all pregnant women as the benefits seem to far outweigh any theoretical and remote risks of vaccination. Government of India has now permitted Covid-19 vaccinations during pregnancy.

29.2: IMMUNIZATION IN LACTATION

Immunization of a lactating mother is expected to benefit the baby as well due to transfer of maternal antibodies through breast milk. However, there is also a potential risk of transfer of vaccine-induced infection. General recommendations for immunization of a lactating mothers are as follows –

- All vaccines are safe in breastfeeding women and pose no harm to the babies, except the yellow fever vaccine.

- Transmission of the yellow fever vaccine virus through breast milk, resulting in infantile meningoencephalitis is known. If unavoidable due to travel compulsions, breastfeeding should be interrupted for the 10 day, after Yellow fever vaccine to escape post-vaccination viremia.

- IAP strongly recommends the administration of COVID-19 vaccines to all breastfeeding women as the real benefits are much more than "theoretical risks" and Government of India has now permitted vaccination of lactating mothers.

Frequently Asked Questions (FAQs)

1. **What was the need to replace previously recommended TT dose during pregnancy with Td (NIS) or Tdap (IAP) doses?**

   Protection against diphtheria and Pertussis from the primary series in infancy wanes overtime. To avoid the accumulation of susceptibles, booster doses of a diphtheria-containing vaccine are needed and hence TT has been replaced with Td in NIS, as per WHO recommendations. IAP suggests that immunization of pregnant women with a single dose of Tdap may be an effective approach to protect very young infants and neonates from Pertussis and hence, it recommended First/only dose of Td to be replaced with Tdap during pregnancy.

2. **Since MMR is contraindicated in pregnancy, whether a woman of reproductive age needs pregnancy test before taking catch-up dose of MMR?**

Routine pregnancy test is not recommended before MMR vaccination

3. **A woman came to know later that she was pregnant while taking a catch-up dose of MMR last week. Whether she must consider termination of pregnancy?**

Termination of pregnancy is not warranted, if the vaccine has been received inadvertently in this period.

4. **Whether pregnant women are at higher risk for complications after Covid vaccines?**

Many covid vaccines have shown potential risk of thromboembolic complications. Since pregnancy is also a period of thrombogenic state, it is unknown whether the risk of thromboembolism increases due to vaccination in pregnancy. However, based on reported risks from general population, this additional risk is likely to be rare and no such reports have emerged.

References

1. Shastri D. Immunization in Special situations. *In:* IAP Guidebook on Immunization 2018-19 - Advisory Committee on Vaccines and Immunization Practices, Indian Academy of Pediatrics, 3rd Edition, New Delhi, Jaypee Brothers 2020; pp 404-432.
2. Mitra M. Vaccination in special situations. *In:* Vashishtha V et al. FAQs on Vaccines and immunization practices. 2nd Edition. New Delhi, Jaypee Brothers 2015; pp 54-62.
3. Immunization in special circumstances. Red Book® 2021-2024 Report of the Committee on Infectious Diseases, American Academy of Pediatrics. Kimberlin Et al (Eds), 32nd Edition, 2021; pg 67-99.

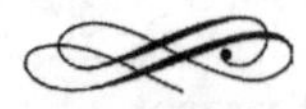

Section

VII

Vaccination In Clinical Practice

Safe Immunization Practices: Counseling, Administration & Pain Control

Immunization is a unique intervention in the sense that the child is otherwise healthy and any error or compromise on the safety may have serious medical, ethical and legal dimensions apart from negative impact on acceptability of immunization programs.

Immunization errors are leading causes of adverse events following immunization (Chapter 6), perhaps more common than the actual side-effects of vaccine products. This chapter deals with important recommendations and suggestions to make immunization a safe event in practice.

30.1: ASSESSING THE NEED AND ELIGIBILITY

All children should be assessed for immunization status at every point of contact, even if they are sick or presented for different reasons. This assessment must –

- Verify the child's age, preferably from the immunization card or by history, if it is not available.

- Verify the vaccines that the child has received till now from the immunization card or by history. Indirect clues e.g. presence of BCG scar, age and site of previous vaccinations, price paid for the same (in private sector) etc. may be used to identify the vaccines received earlier, if required. A new card should be filled out, if the old immunization card is lost or not available.

- Identify all the vaccine/s that the child needs now, including those due for the age and those which were missed in the past. Any recommended immunization schedule – NIS or IAP, may be followed depending on the needs and affordability, after discussing with care-givers.

- Customize the vaccination schedule as per individual requirements and previous immunization status to include missed vaccines (Ch 5.3). All or many required vaccines can be administered during the same session to minimize number of visits (except PCV13 and Menactra®, which should be given at least 4 weeks apart, first being PCV13).

- Assess the contraindications or precautions for due vaccines to determine the eligibility of the child to receive them (**Table 30.1**). *Contraindications* denote the conditions which increase the risk for a serious adverse reaction to vaccination and in such cases the concerned vaccine should not be administered. *Precaution* is a condition which might increase the risk for serious adverse reaction *or* cause diagnostic confusion or compromise the ability of the vaccine to produce immunity. Vaccinations in such cases may proceed with additional care or may be be deferred unless benefits exceed the risk.

- While vaccination is not contraindicated during mild illnesses, it may be deferred in case the care-giver is apprehensive. In such case, they should be advised to return as early as possible for immunization, when the child is well.

- Schedule an immunization appointment on earliest possible date, if not possible on the same day.

30.2: COUNSELLING THE PARENTS

Appropriate communication with parents is key to make them appreciate the need for a vaccine, specially which are not the part of NIS. One-to-one discussion with them on this issue must focus on following points –

- *Factual risk of developing the disease* or its complications in the given population.

- *Efficacy of the vaccine/s* to prevent this disease or its complications in simple terms without raising unrealistic

Table 30.1: Important contraindications & precautions for Common Vacciness[5]		
Vaccine	**Contraindications**	**Precautions**
General	Severe allergic reaction (e.g., anaphylaxis) after previous dose of same vaccine or its component	Moderate or severe acute illness with or without fever
BCG	Severe Immunodeficiency states	–
DTwP/ DTaP/ Tdap	Encephalopathy not attributable to another identifiable cause, within 7 days of previous dose	- Progressive neurologic disorder - GBS within 6 weeks of any TCV - Arthus-type reaction after any TCV (defer vaccination for 10 yrs)
DT/Td	–	- GBS within 6 weeks of any TCV - Arthus-type reaction after any TCV (defer vaccination for 10 years)
HBV	Severe Yeast allergy	–
HiB	Age < 6 weeks	–
IPV	–	Pregnancy
RV	- SCID - History of intussusception	- Immunodeficiency, other than SCID - Chronic GIT disease, Spina bifida or bladder exstrophy
PCV	- Severe allergic reaction to any Diphtheria toxoid containing vaccine - Severe Yeast allergy	–
IIV	–	- GBS < 6 weeks after previous dose - Egg allergy except simple hives
MMR	- Pregnancy - Severe immunodeficiency - Family h/o immunodeficiency	- Recent h/o receiving antibody-containing product (**Table 28.1**) - H/o Thrombocytopenia
JE (Live)	- Severe immunodeficiency - Family h/o immunodeficiency	–
HAV	–	–
Varicella	- Severe immunodeficiency - Pregnancy - Family h/o immunodeficiency	- Recent h/o receiving antibody-containing product (**Table 28.1**) - Antiviral therapy (e.g. acyclovir) in last 24 hrs. Avoid for 14 days after vaccine) - Aspirin Therapy
HPV	Severe Yeast allergy	–
MCV	Severe Yeast allergy	

TCV: Tetanus containing vaccine, **GBS:** Guillan Barre syndrome expectations. It must be clarified that no vaccine is 100% effective and vaccine failures do occur occasionally. However, even in case of such failures, partial protection is expected to reduce the morbidity and complications.

- *Safety of the vaccine* must be emphasized during this session, in realistic terms. All currently used vaccines are very safe but occasional side-effect are not uncommon. It may be emphasized to parents that - a) benefits of vaccination far outweigh the risk of side-effects and b) Most of side-effects are minor, transient and easily manageable.

- *Cost of the vaccine* is an important consideration for parents visiting private sector and should be informed in advance along with available alternatives to let them make an informed decision. Many vaccines have equally effective options (DTaP vs DTwP) but with some differences in side-effects. Some indigenously manufactured vaccines are less expensive but equally effective than imported ones e.g. Rotavirus vaccines. Parents should also be informed regarding free-of-cost availability of some of these vaccines under NIS. They should be made to realize that once accepting a paid vaccine, they may also need to give subsequent doses preferably of the same brands, if required, to avoid late defaults due to cost-factors.

- Parent must also be informed about the scheduling differences for the same vaccine in NIS and IAP recommendations, with logic behind such differences and options.

Appropriate counseling of parents will go a long way to alleviate their fears and apprehensions and ensure proper compliance. However, a written consent is not necessary before vaccination (IAP).

Vaccine hesitancy i.e. the *reluctance or refusal to vaccinate despite the availability* of vaccines has been recognized as one of the leading threats to global health. WHO's Strategic Advisory Group of Experts (SAGE) defines vaccine hesitancy as an individual's behavior, influenced by the 3Cs -*Confidence* i.e.

Trust or no trust in the vaccine or provider; *Complacency* i.e. Perceived need or value of the vaccine, and **C**onvenience i.e. ease or difficulty of access. It is the duty of HCW to identify the reason/s for vaccine hesitancy in care-givers and allay their concerns.

30.3. SAFE INJECTION PRACTICES

All injections involve a breach in the continuity of skin/ mucosa hence, are potentially unsafe, According to a WHO report, nearly 30% of injections used for vaccinations worldwide are unsafe. A safe injection shall not only harm the recipient, but also not expose the provider to avoidable risk or result in a waste that is dangerous to other people. Important recommendations of safe injection practices are as follows –

A. **Hand-washing:** HCW should wash the hands with soap & water, if visibly dirty or may disinfect with an alcohol-based hand rub. Disinfection is also necessary in between the patients during same session. An HCW should avoid giving injections, if suffering from a local infection or cut which may come in contact with injected substance, blood or body fluids. Gloves are not necessary, though single-use gloves may be used and changed between patients, if soiled.

B. **Examine the vaccine product:** Each vaccine vial must be examined for the name, expiry date and batch number mentioned over the label as well as the status of VVM (Ch 4) and date and time of opening the multi-dose vials, if applicable. Similar scrutiny is also necessary for diluents, if applicable.

It is advisable to review the package-insert, even if a vaccine is being used frequently, as specifications are often subject to change. The insert must be checked for - a) Ingredient/s, b) Instructions for reconstitution, c) Dosage & mode of administration, d) Storage instructions to confirm the compliance, and e) warning statements regarding caution and contraindications.

C. **Prepare the vaccine:** While many vaccines are currently available as pre-filled products, many others need to be drawn in a syringe from the single/multi-dose vials or to be reconstituted before use. Following precautions are necessary while preparing a vaccine for administration -

- Vaccine shot must be prepared in a clean designated area where blood or body fluid contamination is unlikely. Multi-dose vials should not be kept in this area to prevent inadvertent contamination.

- All vaccines must be prepared separately for each child and should not be kept as pre-filled syringes in advance.

- Cracks and leaks in vials are not uncommon sources of contamination, which should also be checked for any leakage, pilferage or suspended particles in the contents before use.

- Swabbing the vial-top with antiseptic or disinfectant is not necessary and may itself be the source of contamination. However if necessary, vials may be cleaned with a dry single-use antiseptic swab and not by stored wet-cotton balls.

- Each vaccine must be reconstituted as per manufacturer's recommendations, using *only* the diluents supplied by the manufacturer, if required. Such vaccines should be reconstituted immediately before use.

- Multi-dose vials carry higher risk of contamination and should be used strictly as per *Open-vial Policy* (FAQ 2). Needle used to withdraw the vaccine from this vial should not be left behind in the septum for redrawing, to avoid contamination.

- Whenever possible, vaccine shot must be prepared away from the sight of the child to avoid anxiety.

D. **Positioning the child:** Unexpected motion at the time of injection may injure the child or cause needle-stick injuries to the HCW. Correct positioning with gentle restraining of the child is important to avoid such accidents.

- Child is usually more comfortable in presence of mother or caretaker, who should be permitted to participate in positioning of the child to minimize the anxiety.

- Choice of the position depends on age of the child and site of administration, as suggested in **Fig. 30.1**. While *Cuddling* position or *lying-down* position is preferred for infants, older children may be permitted to sit upright in mother's lap or held in the *straddle* position. School children and adolescents may be immunized sitting upright independently, if cooperative.

- While forcible restraining is not advisable, parent (or an assistant) may tuck the child's legs between theirs to secure them or hold the child's free arm.

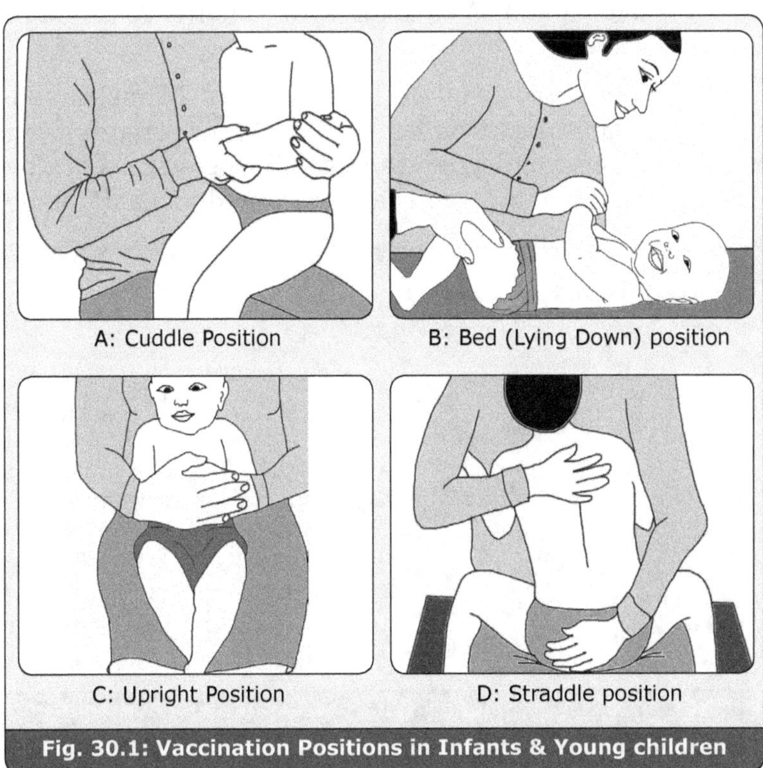

Fig. 30.1: Vaccination Positions in Infants & Young children

- Even though the child is securely positioned and restrained, s/he should be gently informed about the injection.

E) Route of administration: Vaccines are usually administered via intramuscular, subcutaneous or intradermal route (**Fig. 30.2**) as per the manfacturer's instructions or national guidelines, which are not interchangeable and should be strictly followed.

- *Intramuscular (IM) injections* are given by piercing the skin at 90° with a longer 23-24 Gauze needle. All vaccines, containing adjuvants are generally administered IM, due to higher risk of local reactions following superficial injections.

- *Subcutaneous injections* must be administered by pinching up the skin with provider's fingers and piercing it at 45-60°angle with a shorter 23-25 gauze needle.

- *Intradermal injections* e.g. BCG (or ID-rabies) are administered over left shoulder or upper arm using a Tuberculin syringe and small 25 gauze needle, by stretching the skin between non-dominant thumb

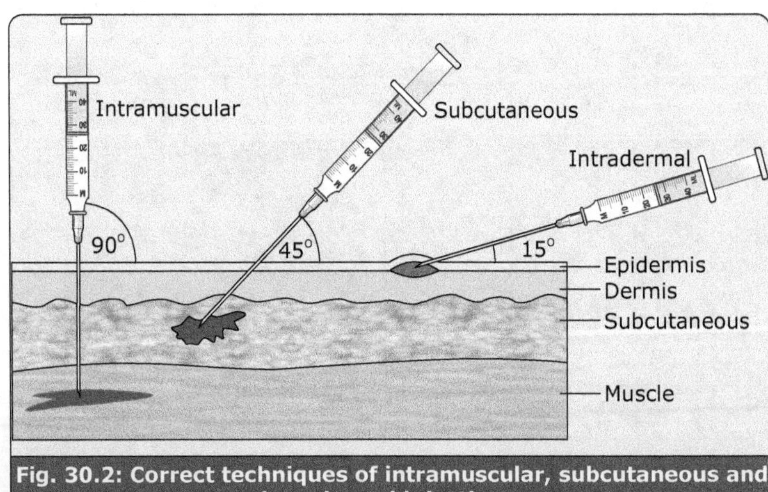

Fig. 30.2: Correct techniques of intramuscular, subcutaneous and intradermal injections.

and fingers and piercing it at ~15° with the bevel of needle facing upwards. Only the needle tip should be introduced beneath the skin. A successful intradermal injection is reflected by formation of a small wheel at the site.

F) **Site of Vaccination:** NIS and other schedules generally specify the recommended sites for each vaccine injection (**Table 5.1**) for the sake of uniformity, which should be adhered to unless the change is warranted due to local causes e.g. infection etc. (**Fig. 30.3**). Using the uniform sites also help to identify vaccines that the child has received as well as the culprit vaccine in case of local adverse event.

- Anterolateral aspect of thigh is the safest and preferred choice for intramuscular injections in infants, in whom upper arm or deltoid region should NOT be used due to inadequate muscle mass. Older children may be administered IM vaccines on upper arm in deltoid region. Vaccinations are usually avoided in highly fatty gluteal region since the antigen deposited in the fat may not invoke appropriate immune response.

- Subcutaneous injections are usually administered over outer aspect of the upper arm, though may be given over thighs in infants.

- Intradermal injections e.g. BCG are given over the shoulder or upper arm, conventionally on left side.

- Two injections must preferably be given on opposite sides, If required in the same sitting, However, more injections can be administered on same site, separated by at least 2.5 cm to avoid overlap of local reactions.

G) **Use of sterile injection equipments:** WHO no longer recommends the use of standard disposable syringes and needles due to risk of potential re-use. Auto disable syringes (**Fig. 30.4**) are preferred for immunization purposes in NIS, manufactured in a way that the plunger cannot be withdrawn after the single use to prevent re-use.

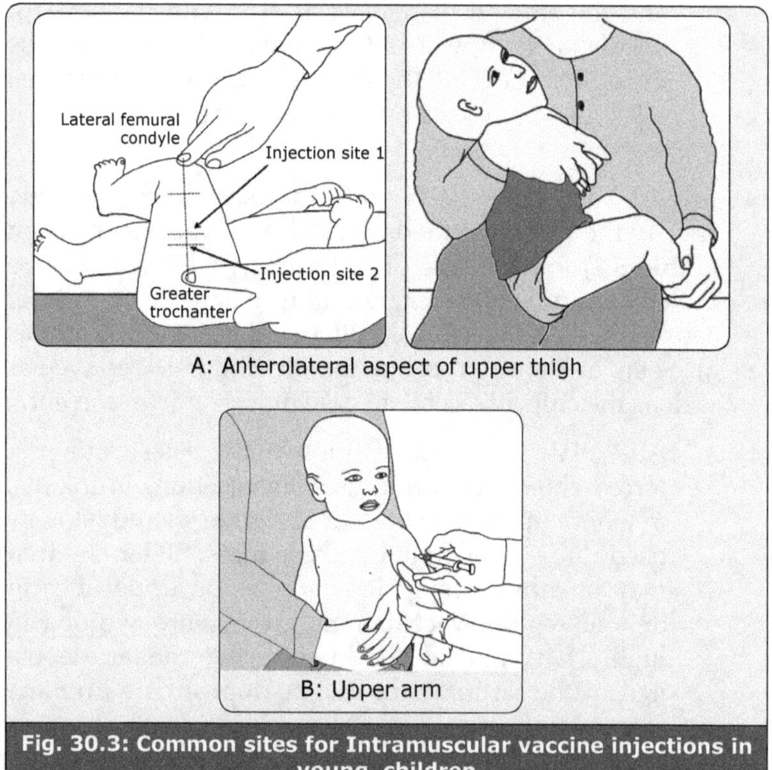

Fig. 30.3: Common sites for Intramuscular vaccine injections in young children

However disposable syringes & needles are frequently used in practice. Some important considerations while using selecting injection instrument are as follows –

- Package containing these syringe and/or needle should be carefully inspected before opening the same and should be discarded, if found to be punctured, torn or damaged.

- Changing needles between drawing vaccine into the syringe and injecting it into the child is not necessary, unless potentially contaminated.

- A longer 23-24 Gauze needle (min 2.5 cm in length) is preferred for Intramuscular injections to reach at

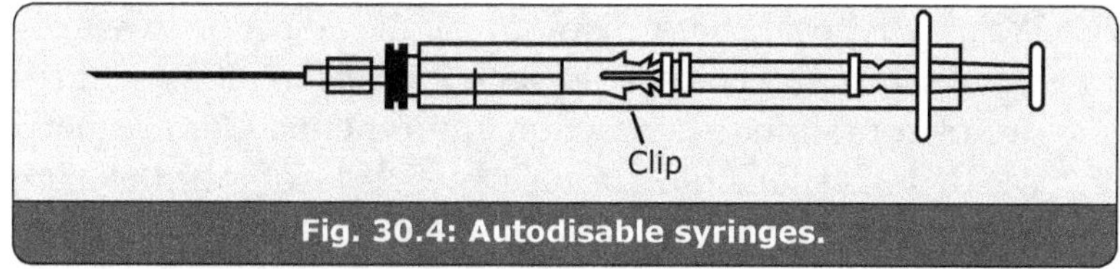

Fig. 30.4: Autodisable syringes.

a deeper tissue plain while shorter needles may be used for subcutaneous or intradermal injections.

- While using an autodisabled syringe, plunger should not be pushed forward before the injection to inject the air in a vial, as this might disable it.

H) **Administering the Injection:** After the child is properly positioned and restrained and the injection is ready, following recommendations must be considered –

- Selected injection site should be inspected for any local infection etc. and must be cleaned with a swab, if dirty. Cotton swabs stored wet in a multi-use container should not be used.

- Vigorous Swabbing of the skin with antiseptic before injection is unnecessary and may add to the anxiety. Organisms colonizing the clean injection site are usually non-pathogenic. However, If an antiseptic swab is used, it should be prepared just before use and product-specific skin contact time must be adhered. Some studies have demonstrated contaminated disinfectant as the source of invasive infection in children.

- No antiseptic swabs should be used for local cleaning before administration of a live vaccine like BCG as it may deactivate pathogens.

- Aspiration i.e. pulling back on the syringe plunger after insertion of the needle but before pushing the liquid is not advised as no large vessels are present at the recommended sites and the process might be more painful for infants due to movement of needle.

I) **Waste disposal:** Safe disposal of the injection waste is essential to prevent needle-stick injuries to HCW and re-use of contaminated injection equipments. Unsafe sharp waste is responsible for nearly 5-28% of needle stick injuries. Following methods are recommended to dispose immunization waste after injection -

- The needle should be cut at the point of use only with a electric or mechanical needle-cutter and disposed-off along with part of the syringe nozzle in the puncture-proof sharps container.

- Remaining part of plastic syringe and vaccine vial must be disposed in the Red bag.

- Empty vaccine vials/ampoules and swabs etc. may be discarded in yellow bags.

- *Recapping* of the used needle is a major cause of needle-stick injuries to the provider, accounting for 25-30% of all needle stick injuries. Ideally, the used needles should be dropped in an enclosed puncture/leak proof sharp's container. However, If recapping is necessary i.e. sharp's container is not available, *Single-handed scooping-re-sheathing technique* may be used to minimize the risk.

i) **Post-vaccination Observation:** All vaccinated cases must be observed for 15-30 minutes after injection for a major adverse event e.g. anaphylaxis. All vaccination sites – fixed or outreach, must be equipped to handle anaphylaxis using anaphylaxis kits (Ch 6.2).

30.4: REDUCING THE PAIN AND ANXIETY

Injectable vaccines are source of significant pain and anxiety which could have a negative influence on the acceptance of further immunizations. However, pain during vaccinations may be mitigated to some extent and managing pain does not decrease the efficacy of the vaccine. Some simple and effective evidence-based strategies to mitigate pain during vaccinations are as follows –

- HCW should be calm, reassuring and well-trained to deal with young kids. Phrases which raise the anxiety e.g. *here comes the sting,* or promote distrust e.g. *it will not hurt or will hurt only for a second,* must be avoided.

- Mother (or care-giver) must be allowed to remain present during vaccination to reassure the child and hold him/her in desired position. Swaddling or sways the child before or after injection by mother may help to comfort the child.

- Infants may be breast-fed during or shortly after the vaccination. There are no reports of adverse effects of breastfeeding during vaccination, including aspiration.

- Feeding small volume of sweet liquids e.g. 1-2 ml Sugar solution before or soon after the injection might help to distract the infant and cope with the discomfort. When rotavirus vaccine is also being given along with other injectable vaccines, it may be given first to have pain-mitigating effect due to sucrose content.

- Distraction measures e.g. toys, video, music, conversation) to divert attention away from pain to something more pleasant are often useful.

- Multiple vaccines, if necessary in same session, must be administered in a sequence, starting with oral ones, then less painful injections e.g. BCG (intradermal) and lastly, more painful IM injections. *WHO recommended sequence of multiple vaccines in same sitting, if required, is as follows – RV > OPV > BCG > Penta V > MR/MMR > JE.*

- Local cooling of the injection site by a topical refrigerant spray immediately before vaccination or application of a topical anesthetic 15-30 minutes before the injection has been proven to reduce the pain though not generally used in mass inmmunization sessions due to logistic issues. There is no evidence that these measures interfere with the immune response.

- Plunger should not be withdrawn after insertion of the needle to aspirate and check for blood as no large vessels are present at recommended sites and the process may cause pain due to longer contact time and lateral movement of the needle.

- Warming the vaccine by rubbing between palms, vigorous rubbing at the injection site or prophylactic administration of an analgesic before injection is not recommended due to lack of evidence of pain-mitigation effectiveness or potential for altering vaccine effectiveness.

- Oral analgesics e.g. paracetamol may be used to mitigate pain and/or fever after the vaccination. However, Studies in children with previous febrile seizures have not demonstrated antipyretics to be effective in the prevention of febrile seizures after vaccination.

Frequently Asked Questions (FAQs)

1. **Parents have lost the immunization card and do not remember giving a particular vaccine? Whether it can be given again?**

   While all efforts should be made to ascertain the receipt of non-receipt of a vaccine, in most cases an additional dose will not cause an adverse event and may be given, within the recommended catch-up period.

2. **What is multi-dose open policy?**

   Multi-dose vials of some vaccines from which one or more doses have been removed, may be used in subsequent immunization sessions for up to **maximum of four weeks**, *provided - a)* The expiry date has not passed, b) The vaccines are stored under appropriate cold-chain conditions, c) The vaccine vial septum has not been submerged in water, d) Aseptic technique has been used to withdraw all doses and e) the VVM, if attached, has not reached the discard point.

This policy does not apply to the vaccines which need to be reconstituted before use e.g. BCG, MR, Yellow fever etc, which should be discarded at the end of session or after 6 hours, whichever is earlier.

3. **Why is the RV vaccine advised to be given before the OPV?**

RV vaccine is preferably given before OPV as it has a larger volume and easier to administer when the infant is most calm.

4. **Why does NIS specify the sides of the body sites to give a vaccine (e.g. Left shoulder for BCG):**

National guidelines specify the sides of the body to which a vaccine must be given for the sake of uniformity and ease of follow-up by surveyors (if the card is lost) *or* identity the culprit vaccine for a local reaction. For example, recommended sides include - BCG on left upper arm, fIPV on Right upper arm, PCV on Right thigh, MR in Right upper arm, JE on Left upper arm etc. However, these sites may be changed in an individual child, in case of any local contraindication e.g. infection etc.

5. **Whether two injections can be given at the same site?**

Yes, If necessary, two injections can be given at same site but with minimum 2.5 cm distance between them.

6. **While preparing a vaccine, diluents ampoule broke accidentally. Can we use any other diluent to reconstitute the vaccine?**

No. Only manufacturer recommended diluents must be used for reconstitution (Ch 2.2).

7. **Why is it not advisable to clean the injection site with a spirit swab before vaccination?**

It is not advisable to use alcohol or spirit swab for local cleaning before live vaccines as some of the live components of the vaccine are killed if they come in contact with spirit.

8. **Why are most of the Intramuscular vaccines not advised to be given over gluteal region?**

    Intramuscular vaccines are avoided over gluteal region to prevent sciatic nerve damage. Moreover, vaccine deposited in the fat of the gluteal region does not invoke the appropriate immune response.

9. **A vaccine was inadvertently given by a route other than the recommended one. What should be done?**

    All precautions should be taken to administer a vaccine by the recommended route only. If by error, live attenuated viral vaccines, which are usually administered subcutaneously have been inadvertently given by the intramuscular route, it need not be repeated. Inadvertent subcutaneous administration of inactivated Hepatitis A vaccine and IPV is also considered valid. For all other vaccines administered by a non–standard route, the dose should be considered invalid and repeated anytime for inactivated vaccines or after at least 4 weeks for live vaccines.

References

1. Ministry of Health and Family welfare, Government of India. Safe injections and waste disposal. *In:* Immunization Handbook for health workers 2018; pp 107-126.
2. World Health organization. Immunization in practice: a practical guide for health staff – 2015 update. Module 3: Ensuring Safe injections. pg 3(3) – 3 (22)
3. World Health organization. Immunization in practice: a practical guide for health staff – 2015 update. Module 5: Managing an immunization session. pg 5 (3) – 3 (34).
4. World Health Organization. Position paper on Reducing pain at the time of vaccination: Weekly Epidemiological Record 2015 (Sept);39:505-510.
5. Kroger A et al. General Best Practice Guidelines for Immunization (updated May 4 2021). Available at *https://www.cdc.gov/vaccines/hcp/acip-recs/general-recs/index.html* (accessed on 18th May 2021).
6. Pemde HK. Practical aspects of Immunization. *In:* IAP Guidebook on Immunization 2018-19 - Advisory Committee on Vaccines and Immunization Practices, Indian Academy of Pediatrics, 3rd Edition, New Delhi, Jaypee Brothers 2020; pp 39-49.

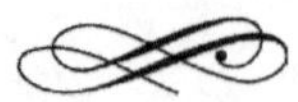

Vaccines at a Glance (Available in India)

Vaccines (Brands)	Dose & Route of Administration	Immunization Schedule (with upper age limit)		Efficacy	Adverse Events	Contraindi-cation
		NIS	IAP			
BCG[LF] (*Tubervac*)	0.1 ml ID (0.05 ml<1 mo)	Birth **(Upto 1 Yr)**	Birth **(Upto 5 Yr)**	50-60% 70-90% for severe disease	Lymphadenitis Diss. TB	IDD
HBV (*Engerix, Genevac-B, Bevac, Revac B*)	0.5 ml IM (1 ml >18 yr)	Birth, 6, 10, 14 wk **(Upto 1 Yr)**	Birth, 6, 10, 14 weeks (Last dose not < 24 wk or <16 wk of first dose) **(No age limit)** 0.1.6 mo	>95%	NS	None
bOPV[L] (*Biopolio B1/3, Biomed-Polio*)	2 drops PO	Birth, 6, 10, 14 wk, B: 16-24 mo	Birth dose only	~100%	VAPP/VDPV	IDD
IPV (*Polyprotec, Poliovac, Imovax Polio*)	0.5 ml IM/SC 0.1 ml ID (in NIS)	6, 14 wk (as fIPV) **(Upto 1 Yr)**	6, 10, 14 weeks B: 15-18 mo, 5-6 yrs **(No age limit)**	95-100%	NS	None
HiB[F (some brands)] (*Hiberix, Bio-Hib, Peda-Hib*)	0.5 ml IM (1 ml >18 yr)	6, 10, 14 weeks **(Upto 1 Yr)**	6, 10, 14 weeks B 12-18 mo **(Upto 5 yr)** <12 mo: 2 doses at 0, 1 mo, B 12-18 mo, 12-15 mo: SD, B after 8 weeks > 15 mo: Single dose	>90%	NS	None

For abbreviations used, see last page of appendix

(Continued)

Vaccines (Brands)	Dose & Route of Administration	Immunization Schedule (with upper age limit)		Efficacy	Adverse Events	Contraindi-cation
DTwP (*Triple Antigen, Comvac-3, Tripavac*)	0.5 ml IM	6, 10, 14 wk, B: 16-24 mo, 5 yr **(Upto 1 Yr)**	6, 10, 14 weeks, B: 15-18 mo, 4-5 yrs **(Upto 7 yr)** 0, 1, 6 mo	> 95% for D & T 70-80% for P	Local reactions, Fever, Persistent cry, HHE, Seizures, Encaphalopathy, Anaphylaxis	Encephalopathy Anaphylaxis
DTaP (*Infanrix*)	0.5 ml IM	-	6, 10, 14 weeks, B: 15-18 mo, 4-5 yrs **(Upto 7 yr)** 0, 1, 6 mo	> 95% for D & T 70-80% for P		
Tdap (*Boosterix, Adacel*)	0.5 ml IM	-	SD at 10-12 years SD after 7 yr (if not immunized earlier) SD in each Pregnancy	> 95% for D & T 70-80% for P	None	
DT (*Dual Antigen*)	0.5 ml IM	Alternative to DTwP, If contraindicated	Alternative to DTwP/DTaP, if contraindicated	> 95% for D & T	NS	None
Td (*Sii-Td-Vac, BeTd*)	0.5 ml IM	Booster:10 & 16 yrs Each Pregnancy Wound care	2nd/3rd dose after Tdap (for catch-up DPT immunization > 7 yrs) Wound care	95-100%	NS	None
DTwP+HIB+HBV (*Easy-five, Comvac-5, Pentavac, ComBE Five*)	0.5 ml IM	6, 10, 14 weeks	6, 10, 14 weeks	As for constituent vaccines		
DTaP+HIB+HBV (*Pentaxim*)	0.5 ml IM	-	6, 10, 14 weeks			
DTwP+HIB+HBV+IPV (*Easy-six*)	0.5 ml IM		6, 10, 14 weeks			

For abbreviations used, see last page of appendix

(Continued)

Vaccines (Brands)	Dose & Route of Administration	Immunization Schedule (with upper age limit)		Efficacy	Adverse Events	Contraindication
DTaP+HIB+HBV+IPV (*Hexaxim, Infanrix-Hexa*)	0.5 ml IM		6, 10, 14 weeks			
DTwP+HIB (*Quadravax, Easy4, Tetraxim*)	0.5 ml IM	-	6, 10, 14 weeks, B 15-18 mo			
DTaP+HIB+IPV (*Infanrix-IPV*)	0.5 ml IM	-	6, 10, 14 weeks, B 15-18 mo			
DTwP+HBV (*Comvac-4*)	0.5 ml IM	-	6, 10, 14 weeks			
RV1[LF] (*Rotarix*)	RV1 1 ml,	-	6,, 14 weeks (Two doses) **(first dose not after 15 wks, complete by 32 weeks)**	50-60% 80% for SRVGE	Intussusception	H/O Intussusception SCID
RV5[L] (*Rotateq*)	2 ml PO	-	6,, 14 weeks (Three doses) **(first dose not after 15 wks, complete by 32 weeks)**			
BRV-PV[LF] (*Rotasiil*)	2 ml PO	-				
RHBV1[L] (*Rotavac, Rotasure*)	0.5 ml PO	-				
RHBV1 (D)[L] (*Rotavac-5D*)	5 drops	6, 10, 14 wk **(Upto 1 Yr)**	-			

For abbreviations used, see last page of appendix

(Continued)

Vaccines (Brands)	Dose & Route of Administration	Immunization Schedule (with upper age limit)		Efficacy	Adverse Events	Contraindi-cation
PCV13 (*Prevenar*)	0.5 ml IM (1 ml> 18 yr)	6, 10 wk, 9 mo **(Upto 1 Yr)**	6, 10, 14 weeks, B at 12-15 mo **(Upto 5 yr)** 6-12 mo: 0, 1 mo, B in 2nd yr 12-23 mo: 0.2 mo 23-59 mo: Single dose	> 60-80% (25-35% for Pneumonia, Otitis)	Seizures, HHE	None
PCV10 (*Synflorix, Pneumosiil*)	0.5 ml IM (1 ml> 18 yr)	6, 10 wk, 9 mo **(Upto 1 Yr)**	6, 10, 14 weeks, B at 12-15 mo **(Upto 5 yr)** 6-12 mo: 0, 1 mo, B in 2nd yr 12-59 mo: 0.2 mo	> 60-80% (25-35% for Pneumonia, Otitis)	Seizures, HHE	None
PPSV (*Pneumovax 23*)	0.5 ml IM/SC (1 ml> 18 yr)	-	**In High-risk cases only, with PCV only** SD at 2 yr, Repeat once after 3-5 yr	Uncertain	None	None
MRLF (*MR-Vac, MR(BE)*)	0.5 ml SC (1 ml> 18 yr)	9 mo & 12-15 mo	-	M: 80-95% R: 95-99%	Rash, TCP, Arthralgia, SSPE? TSS*	IDD, pregnancy
MMRLF (*Tresivac, Priorix*)	0.5 ml SC (1 ml> 18 yr)	-	9 mo, 15 mo, 4-6 yrs	M: 80-95% R: 95-99% Mumps: ~90%	As for MR + Parotitis Aseptic meningitis	IDD, pregnancy

For abbreviations used, see last page of appendix   *(Continued)*

Vaccines (Brands)	Dose & Route of Administration	Immunization Schedule (with upper age limit)		Efficacy	Adverse Events	Contraindi-cation
MMRV[LF] (*Priorix-Tetra*)	0.5 ml SC	-	4-6 yr (alternative to second MMR+V) Not to use >12 years	As per component Vaccines,		
Rubella[LF] (*R-Vac*)	0.5 ml SC	-	Rarely used	R: 95-99%	Arthralgia	IDD, pregnancy
J Encephalitis[LF] (*LAV*)	0.5 ml SC	Two doses at 9-12 mo, 16-24mo **(Upto 15 yr)**	-	40-70%	NS	None
J Encephalitis (Inactivated) (*JENVAC*)	SC 0.5 ml	-	Two doses 0, 1 mo after first year **(Upto 18 yr)**	>90%	NS	None
J Encephalitis Inactivated (*JEEV*)	SC 0.5 ml (IM 0.25 ml < 3 yr	-	Two doses 0, 1 mo after first year **(Upto 18 yr)**	>90%	NS	None
TCV (*Typbar-TCV, Zyvac-TCV, Typhibev, Pedatyph, Enteroshield*)	IM/SC 0.5 ml	-	SD 6-9 mo **(Upto 18 yr)**	>98%	NS	None
TPSV (*Typhirix, Typbar, Bio-typh, Vactyph*)	IM/SC 0.5 ml	-	(only if TCV is not available) SD at 2 yr, repeat every 3 yr **(Upto 18 yr)**	55-70% for 2-3 yr	NS	None

For abbreviations used, see last page of appendix

(Continued)

Vaccines (Brands)	Dose & Route of Administration	Immunization Schedule (with upper age limit)		Efficacy	Adverse Events	Contraindi-cation
HAV (Inactivated) (*Havrix, Havpur, Avaxim*)	IM 0.5 ml (1 ml > 19 yr)	-	Two doses after 1 yr, at 6-18 mo interval **(Upto 10 yr/>10 yr after screening)**	90-95%	NS	None
HAV (LAV)[LF] (*Biovac-A*)	SC 0.5 ml	-	SD (1-15 yrs) **(Upto 10 yr/>10 yr after screening)**	100%	NS	IDD
HAV+HBV (*Twinrix*)	IM 0.5 ml	=	0, 1, 6 months	As per constituent vaccines		
Varicella[L] (*Varilrix, Varivax, Okavax*)	SC 0.5 ml	-	Two doses at 15 mo and after 3-6 mo (Dose interval 6 weeks in High-risk cases)	70-90% (>99% for severe disease)	MVLI, Breakthrough V, H zoster-	IDD, pregnancy, Salicylate Rx
Influenza (inactivated) (*Fluquadri, Vaxiflu-4, Fluarix-Tetra, Influvac_tetra*)	IM/SC 0.5 ml (0.25 ml < 3 yr for some brands)	-	2 doses 0.4 wks at mo > SD annualy **(Normally Upto 5 years)** *High-risk cases* <9yr:Two doses 0.4 wks > SD annually > 9 yr: SD annually	59% 36% for ILI	Fberile seizures, GBS	H/O GBS
Influneza[L] **(Live)** (*Nasovac-S*)	0.25 ml in each nostril	-	SD annually after 2 yr age	82% 33% for ILI	Flu-like illness	IDD

For abbreviations used, see last page of appendix

(Continued)

Vaccines (Brands)	Dose & Route of Administration	Immunization Schedule (with upper age limit)		Efficacy	Adverse Events	Contraindi-cation
HPV2 (*Cervarix*)	IM 0.5 ml	-	9-15 yr: Two doses at 0.6 mo 15-26 yr: Three doses at 0, 1, 6 mo	~ 90% Pre-can: 75% Warts: 30-50%	NS	Pregnancy
HPV4 (*Gardasil*)	IM 0.5 ml	-	99-15 yr: Two doses at 0.6 mo 15-26 yr: Three doses at 0, 2, 6 mo			
MCV (*Menactra*)	IM 0.5 ml	-	**In High-risk cases only** (9 mo-55 yr) 9-23 mo: Two doses at 0, 3 mo >2 yr: SD B every 5 yrs (every 3 yr < 7 yr age)	96-100%	NS, ? GBS	H/o GBS
MCV (*Menveo*)	IM 0.5 ml	-	**In High-risk cases only** (2 yr-55 yr) Single dose Not licensed < 2 yr in India B every 5 yrs			

For abbreviations used, see last page of appendix

(Continued)

Vaccines (Brands)	Dose & Route of Administration	Immunization Schedule (with upper age limit)		Efficacy	Adverse Events	Contraindi-cation
MPSVF (*Quadrimeningo*)	SC 0.5 ml	-	**In High-risk cases only, if MCV NA** SD after 2 yr, repeat every 3-5 yr **Outbreak** 3-24 mo: Two doses at 3 mo interval >24 mo: SD	>85%	GIT upset, LN+	None
Cholera (*Shancol*)	PO 1.5 ml	-	**In High-risk cases only** Two doses at 2 wk interval Booster after 2 yr, if required	~65%	GIT upset	None
Yellow Fever[LF] (*Stamaril*)	0.5 ml SC/IM		**Travellers to endemic countries** After 6 mo age: SD 10 days before travel	>90%	YELAND, YELAVD	Egg allergy, Pregnancy
Rabies (PCEV)[F] (*Rabipur, Vaxirab-N, Chirorab*)	IM 1 ml ID 0.1 ml	-	PEP: IM D 0, 3, 7, 21-28 ID D 0, 3, 7, 30 (Two site/visit) PrEP: IM/ID D 0 & 7 Re-PEP*: IM/ID D 0 & 3	>99%	NS	Severe egg allergy
Rabies (PDEV)[F] (*Vaxirab*)	IM 1 ml ID 0.1 ml	-			None	
Rabies (PVRV)[F] (*Abhayrab, Verorab, Indirab, Berab, Rabivax-S, Zuvirab, Zoonovac-V*)	IM (0.5 ml ID 0.1 ml	-				
Rabies (HDCV)[F] (*Imovax-Ravies*)	IM 1 ml (not for ID use)	-	PEP: D 0, 3, 7, 21-28 PrEP: D 0 & 7 RePEP*: D 0 & 3		Headache, Allergy	

Abbreviations: **B**: Booster, **F (superscript)**: Freeze-dried vaccine, **ID**: Intradermal, **IDD**: Immunodeficiency disorders, **IM**: Intramuscular, **L (superscript)**: Live attenuated vaccine, **MO**: Month, **MVLI**: Modified varicella like illness, **NS**: Not Significant, **PO**: Per oral, **SCID**: Severe combined Immunodeficiency, **SD**: Single dose, **SSPE**: Subacute sclerosing panencephalirtis, **TCP**: Thrombocytopenia, **TSS**: Toxic Shock Syndrome, **Wk**: Week/s, **Yr**: Year, **YELAND**: *Yellow fever vaccine-associated neurologic disease*, **YEVAND**: *Yellow fever vaccine-associated viscerotropic disease*

Note: f and t refer to figures and tables respectively.

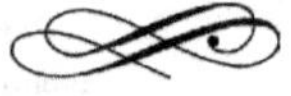